feel
confident

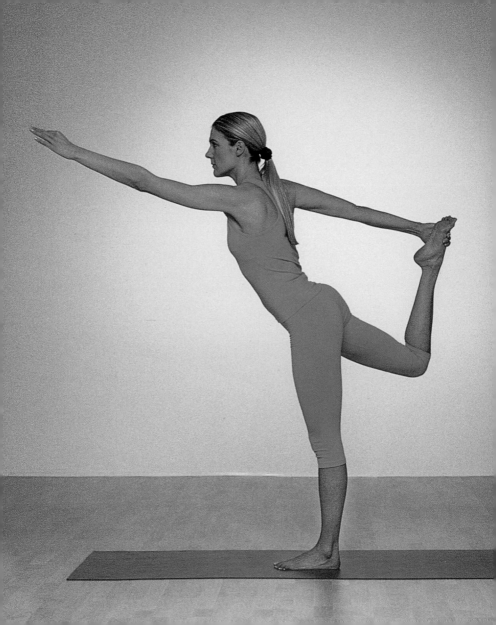

feel
confident

Uma Dinsmore-Tuli

YOGA BIOMEDICAL TRUST

DK Publishing

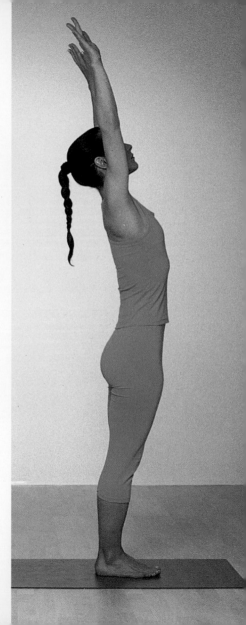

London, New York, Munich,
Melbourne, and Delhi

Series art editor: Anne-Marie Bulat
Series editor: Jane Laing

Series consultant: Peter Falloon-Goodhew
Managing editor: Gillian Roberts
Senior art editor: Karen Sawyer
Category publisher: Mary-Clare Jerram

US editor: Maggi McCormick
DTP designer: Sonia Charbonnier
Production controller: Joanna Bull

Photographer: Graham Atkins-Hughes
(represented by A & R Associates)

First American Edition, 2002

02 03 04 05 10 9 8 7 6 5 4 3 2 1

Published in the United States by
DK Publishing, Inc.
375 Hudson Street
New York, New York 10014

ISBN: 0-7894-8906-6

Color reproduced in Singapore by
Colourscan
Printed and bound in Hong Kong / China by
South China Printing Co.

See our complete product line at
www.dk.com

contents

introduction

To practice yoga is to develop self-awareness on a physical, mental, and emotional level. Such awareness offers liberation from low self-esteem and a firm foundation on which to build self-confidence.

Practicing yoga gives you the time and the techniques to become aware of aspects of yourself that you tend to overlook in everyday life. At a physical level, yoga teaches you to be aware of your breathing patterns, and of areas of tension or tiredness in your muscles and joints. At a mental and emotional level, yoga helps you to notice your patterns of thought, to be aware of the effects of your attitudes and habits, and to understand your worries and concerns. Yoga is a practical tool that helps you to become self-aware.

This self-awareness is the basis of self-respect. When you begin to respect yourself, you start to build your self-confidence. Yoga nourishes and strengthens the body, mind, and spirit. In practicing it regularly, you will become more aware of your real needs, and grow to recognize your own abilities, attitudes, preferences,

HEALTH CONCERNS

If a health practitioner has advised you not to over-exert yourself physically, or if you have any other health concerns, seek advice from a qualified yoga therapist or teacher (see p.128) before using this book. Page 17 provides basic advice for some common medical conditions and, where appropriate, "Take Care" advice or alternatives are given for individual practices. If you are pregnant, or have recently given birth, ask a suitably qualified yoga teacher which practices would be appropriate for you.

and habits. Yoga promotes confidence and assuredness, enabling you to be comfortable and at ease with yourself. It gives unlimited access to the relaxed and respectful understanding that underpins self-confidence.

Unlike some forms of exercise, yoga is suitable for everyone. Whatever your age or level of fitness, yoga is a very safe form of exercise, provided you work within your limits. However, please read through the text in the box below left, entitled "Health Concerns," before you begin, as some yoga practices can be physically demanding.

Causes of low self-esteem

All too often the erosion of confidence and self-esteem begins with unfavorable comparisons with other people or with some idealized, unrealistic notion of who you think you are or ought to be. Then the spiral of self-criticism and self-recrimination begins, and you lose touch with the reality of your own strengths and weaknesses. You build for yourself a punishing self-image based on harsh expectations.

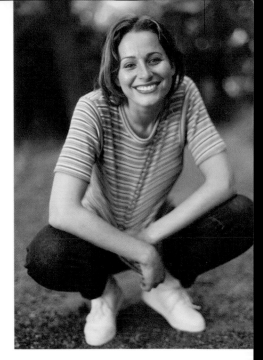

Vitality, good health, and emotional wellbeing are all rooted in the easeful self-confidence that yoga practice develops.

You may come to feel permanently anxious and dissatisfied: everything you do or say, even the way you sleep and eat, does not feel good enough. This is a debilitating burden to carry around with you everywhere, and although your lack of confidence may be psychological and emotional, it can manifest its heaviness in many physical symptoms.

DEALING WITH OTHER PEOPLE'S BEHAVIOR

Sometimes it may appear that the cause of poor self-confidence is another person or the relationship that you have with another person. It is true that there are certain individuals in whose company you may feel buoyant and confident, and others whose very presence makes you feel nervous and inadequate. But this is not to say that other people hold the key to your own self-confidence. You must find your own inner ease and balance, so that you can meet with equilibrium whatever responses you receive in daily life.

If you are involved in relationships with people who persistently seem to make you feel bad about yourself, you owe it to yourself to explore the reasons for this. It may be that you cannot practically avoid dealing with these people, and so you need to learn how to return always to your sense of inner strength and balance in your interactions with them. It may be also that you need to find ways to end relationships that are truly harmful, or in which the power imbalances are severely damaging. While yoga is a valuable help during such change, you may also need the support of a counselor or therapist to address these issues.

For example, you may begin to assume poor sitting or standing postures, or you may be uncomfortable when you lie down to rest. If your body remains in a state of constant discomfort and tension for long enough, your self-confidence can become further eroded, blocking energy, making you tired, irritable, and cross with yourself.

Low energy levels can also be related to poor nutrition and inadequate breathing. Poor breathing habits can also make it hard to maintain concentration. A distracted mind is characterized by an inability to remain in the present and can become full of self-deprecatory fears and self-accusatory anxieties that may be projected into the future. These kinds of thoughts are every bit as dangerous to self-esteem as the tyrant of negative self-image.

There are a number of lifestyle habits that can erode self-esteem. Over-consumption of caffeine can reduce your ability to concentrate and impair your sleep, leading to self-criticism and depression. The use of nicotine, alcohol, marijuana, and other recreational drugs can make it difficult to be honest with yourself, and without real honesty there can be no firm ground for self-confidence. It is worth investigating the rhythms and patterns of your daily life to check for unnecessary and avoidable items of conflict, stress, and energy depletion that can diminish your sense of self-worth. For example, maybe that exhausting daily 10-minute ride in a bus crammed with bad-tempered commuters could be more productively replaced with an enjoyable 30-minute walk?

How yoga can help

Kindness is the best first aid for a wounded self-image. Compassionate awareness gives you freedom from the dictates of negative self-image because it helps you to recognize what really is the best and most comfortable way for you to be. By consistent repetition of some simple yoga practices, you can effectively reinforce the habit of kindly self-awareness that will eventually eradicate the root causes of self-recrimination and poor self-esteem.

The yoga practices in this book all use breath as a way to understand and develop the interaction between body, mind, and emotions. The practices teach how the focus of your mind can alter your breath, and how the change in the breath can help you to communicate more intelligently with your body. Once the body begins to respond, you enter a "positive feedback loop": the sense of wellbeing that you experience physically has a profound impact upon your emotional and mental states. These in turn influence your breath, which promotes a further deepening into ease with the physical body, which makes you feel even better about yourself.

It is an expanding spiral of joy that is deeply practical and very simple. It works to counter the downward spirals of depression and poor self-image, and creates an openhearted ease of confidence and positive self-image that is transformatory. Others notice the positive benefits of your yoga practice and are more positive in their behavior to you, affirming your transformation from without.

The four essential qualities

The yoga practices in this book are designed to promote ease, develop balance, build strength, and sharpen focus. They work with the physical body and breath to access the calm confidence that comes from a more gentle way of living.

Promoting ease

At the heart of a healthy sense of self-confidence is an ease with yourself, a sense of compassion for who you are. To mobilize the energy and strength that comes from developing balance, strength, and focus, you need to establish a comforting confidence in understanding who you are.

Above all, the practice of Full Yogic Breath promotes ease. It helps you to unlearn poor breathing habits, and allows you to take full advantage of the lungs' capacity to draw in vitality and confidence with every breath. When you use this practice in your yogic poses, you release farther and deeper into the work of self-transformation, and build stronger foundations for self- esteem. When you focus on the exhalation in the Humming Breath, you tell yourself you can be easeful and relaxed with who you are. Resting in this ease is the time to let destructive habits and self-criticism pass away, and to use the sound vibrations to nurture and nourish the newly emerging, confident, and powerful self. The relaxation poses – Corpse and Reverse Corpse – together with Resting Crocodile and Hare all teach you about surrender and easeful rest in the moment.

Developing balance

Without steady balance there is no firm ground from which to develop a sense of self-worth. When you have balance, you can be still or move with poise, reflecting a balanced state of mind and emotions.

You can work toward mental and emotional equanimity by developing coordinated balance in the physical body, by linking the breath with the body, and by learning to maintain physical poise in positions that you would not have to do in everyday life (for example, when you stand on your head or shoulders). When you develop balance in your body through yoga, you are better able to withstand the challenges and difficulties of life.

Alternate Nostril Breath, Psychic Triangle Breath, and the Breath Balancing pose all teach how to become self-observant, attentive, and patient as you notice a slow but steady change. These practices

develop wonder and compassion, for every inhalation and every exhalation links us to the source of life, and to the potential for unbounded confidence, power, and trust.

The more physically demanding balances such as Headstand, Tree, and Dancer require and promote clarity of purpose and perseverance. It takes consistent repetition to master

YOGA PRACTICES FOR THE FOUR QUALITIES

The four qualities of ease, balance, strength, and focus together will help you develop self-confidence. The key postures

promoting each quality are listed below. An easeful and balanced foundation is the basis for strength and focus.

Ease

Corpse (see p.19)
Full Yogic Breath (see p.23)
Resting Crocodile (see p.54)
Hare (see p.74)
Spinal Twist & Spinal Twist 2 (see p.90, 92)
Humming Breath (see p.98)

Balance

Yogic Rock and Roll (see p.29)
Tree (see p.40)
Dancer (see p.42)
Snake (see p.52)
Camel (see p.68)
Headstand (see p.86)
Alternate Nostril Breathing (see p.95)
Psychic Triangle Breath (see p.94)
Breath Balancing (see p.99)

Strength

Stirring the Pot (see p.32)
Triangle (see p.38)
Boat (see p.44)
Stoking the Fire (see p.96)
Shining the Skull (see p.97)
Invocation of Energy (see p.100)

Focus

Bow and Arrow (see p.36)
Thunderbolt (see p.62)
Philosopher (see p.64)
Roaring Lion (see p.66)
Concentrated Gazing (see p.102)
Gesture of Consciousness (see p.104)
Gesture of Knowledge (see p.105)
Inner Silence Meditation (see p.106)
Deep Relaxation (see p.108)

these postures, but in practicing them, you develop the clarity of focus to see through negative self-image, and build the perseverance necessary to grow surely in self-confidence.

Building strength

The power to remain poised and balanced in self-esteem requires strength. The strength to remain balanced is a supple strength that enables you to adapt to situations while retaining the power to stand your ground if necessary. The core of physical strength is in the abdomen: the abdominal muscles support the work of the back muscles to hold you upright, and the "fire in your belly" generates the energy for you to accomplish what you need to do.

The most effective yogic practices for developing abdominal strength are the breathing practices Shining the Skull and Stoking the Fire. Combined with Boat, Triangle, and Stirring the Pot, they enable you to develop a core of strength that is truly empowering. When you then practice the Invocation of Energy, you can understand that the world is full of powerful energy available to give, take, and share with each other.

Sharpening focus

Clarity of focus is crucial to self-esteem. To feel confident in yourself, you need to be able to focus both within and without. Internal focus is necessary to understand clearly your

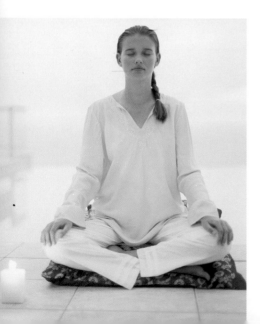

As you develop physical strength and balance, you acquire the emotional equilibrium to feel truly confident.

strengths and weaknesses, and to be compassionate about yourself. External focus is necessary so that you can respond effectively to the situations in which you find yourself, whatever they may be.

Using the focus of the eye in yoga postures helps to sharpen the focus of the mind's eye, to develop clarity of purpose that is at the heart of self-confidence. It is the practice of Concentrated Gazing that most simply and directly teaches the single-pointed gaze. Although, for the most part, the focus of the gaze is an external object, for some of the time the eyes are closed, allowing the inner eye to develop its capacities, too. The Inner Silence Meditation develops this capacity still further, strengthening the concentration of your attention.

The elegant sitting poses – Thunderbolt and Philosopher – provide a physical expression for the focusing of attention, while the simple mudras, or hand gestures, provide subtle but profound physical signs that give further encouragement for the settling of the mind into concentrated awareness.

HOW TO USE THIS BOOK

The remainder of this book is divided into three sections. The **Foundations** section provides guidance on doing yoga and some basic breathing and preliminary stretches. Familiarize yourself with them first before moving on to the **Building Blocks** section. This contains a selection of postures and breathing practices, as well as a simple meditation and relaxation technique. Work through these postures gradually, selecting one or two to work on at a time, rather than trying to do them all at once. Look at the photographs first to get a feel for the overall shape of the posture. Then follow the accompanying step-by-step instructions carefully. If you find a posture difficult to do, work on the preliminary steps first or try the alternative, if one is given.

The **Programs** section combines selected postures and other practices in a series of short yoga programs designed for particular situations and needs. Make sure that you understand how to do the postures first before trying these programs.

Yoga is traditionally learned from a teacher, and you will benefit from going to a class, if you are not already doing so. Organizations that can help you find a qualified teacher are listed on page 128.

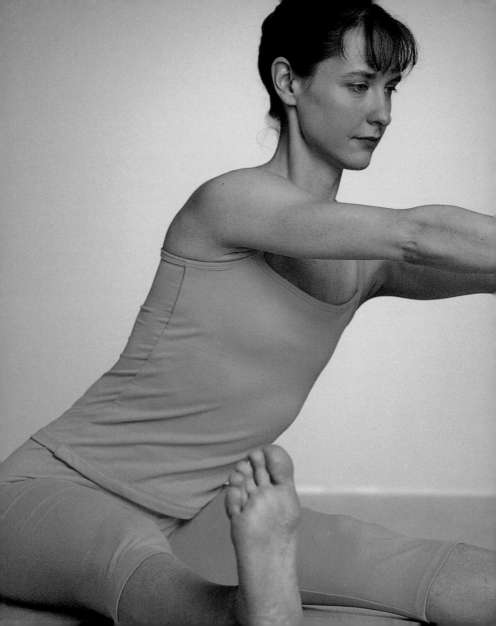

foundations

This section provides advice for those new to yoga. It includes some basic standing, sitting, and lying positions, together with advice on using props. It also contains breath-with-movement exercises to loosen the body and help you deepen the connection with the breath.

before you
start

To develop healthy self-confidence, be guided in your yoga practice by ease and comfort. Do not set yourself unrealistic goals, and practice with focus and concentration, moving with the breath.

Regular and sustained practice is important – a little and often is far better than lengthy sessions with long gaps in between. Be realistic about your available time. It is far more conducive to the development of self-esteem to set yourself the target of a five-minute daily practice, and to meet that target with ease, than to punish yourself because you were unable to practice for half an hour a day. Build up the length of your yoga sessions slowly and you will feel your self-confidence grow.

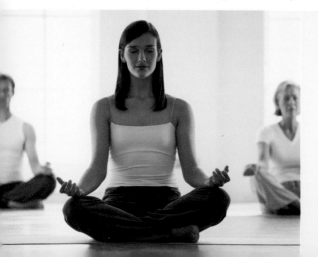

JOINING A CLASS
Practicing yoga regularly in a class with the expert guidance of an experienced yoga teacher can be invaluable when building self-confidence. Making such a commitment can help you develop your skills and abilities, and enhance the qualities of relaxation and ease. In addition, mutual respect between student and teacher promotes self-esteem.

Practice on a mat or other nonslip surface, such as a carpet, and wear loose clothing that allows you to move freely and easily.

Let every breath you take guide you into a compassionate awareness of the needs of your own body. Respect those needs. Never push your body into discomfort or strain.

Work to develop your ability to come into and out of the postures with the same grace, elegance, and dignity as you hold them. Understand that the final form of the posture is the central moment of pause in the flow into and out of the pose.

Support from a teacher

It can be a great boost to self-confidence to attend a yoga class. However, it is important to choose a class with care. Get recommendations from people whose opinions you respect, and whose reasons for doing yoga resonate with your own. Take references from reputable yoga training organizations (see p.128) for qualified teachers in your area, and try as many classes as you need until you find one that you enjoy.

ADVICE FOR COMMON MEDICAL CONDITIONS

• If you have high blood pressure (HBP), a heart condition, glaucoma, or a detached retina, do not let your head stay below your heart.
• If you have HBP or a heart condition, hold strong standing and prone postures for a short time only. In addition, for HBP, keep your arms below your head.
• If you have low blood pressure (LBP), come up slowly from inverted poses.
• If you have a back problem or sciatica, avoid bending and twisting movements that provoke pain or other symptoms (for example, tingling or numbness in the leg). Keep your knees bent in forward bends.
• If you have a hernia, or have had recent abdominal surgery, do not put strong pressure on the abdomen.
• If you have arthritis, mobilize joints to their maximum pain-free range, but rest them if they are inflamed.
• If you have arthritis of the neck or other neck problems, do not tilt the head back in back bends, and be cautious with sideways and twisting neck movements.
• During menstruation, you may need to practice more gently. Avoid inversions and postures that put strong pressure on the pelvic area.

the basics

In yoga, basic standing, sitting, and lying-down positions are important in their own right, helping you develop stability and awareness of the benefits of alignment for your posture, your breathing, and for the free flow of energy. They also provide the foundations from which other postures are developed.

In addition, being able to sit comfortably and steadily is important for breathing practices and also for meditation, helping you remain focused without distractions from physical tensions. Lying down is often used to develop body and breath awareness, and to relax and allow

your body to absorb the beneficial effects of other yoga practices.

If you find it impossible to achieve the full posture, it can be very helpful to use a prop, such as a block or cushion, to make sure you do not strain your body.

STANDING

Stand up straight with your feet parallel, hip-width apart, and your ears, tops of shoulders, hips, and ankles in line. Press your feet into the ground and lift up through your body. Broaden across the top of the chest. Feel balanced in all directions, your head as if suspended by a thread from the ceiling. Look straight ahead, relax, and breathe easily.

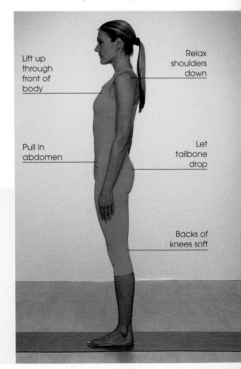

Lift up through front of body

Relax shoulders down

Pull in abdomen

Let tailbone drop

Backs of knees soft

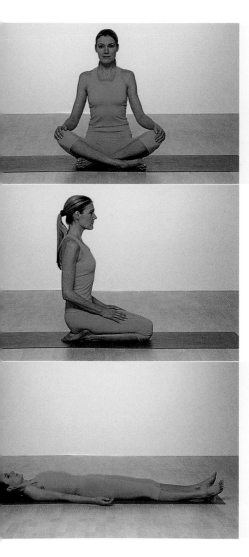

EASY SITTING

This basic posture is good for breathing practices. Cross your shins with the feet under the opposite knee. Position yourself on the front edge of your sitting bones, with the spine long and the head erect. Allow the hips to relax. If your knees are higher than your hips, sit on a block or another support.

KNEELING

Try this position if you find basic cross-legged sitting uncomfortable. Sit on your heels with the tops of your thighs facing the ceiling. Alternativey, if you are going to stay longer, position your knees and feet hip-width apart and sit on blocks, a folded blanket, or a bolster. Keep your spine long and head erect. Rest your hands on your thighs or in your lap.

LYING

Lie on your back to relax at the end of a session or between postures. Lie with your legs stretched out, hip-width apart, feet and legs relaxing out, arms away from your sides, and backs of the hands on the floor. Rest the center of the back of the head on the floor. If you feel any discomfort in your lower back, bend your knees. This is known as Corpse pose.

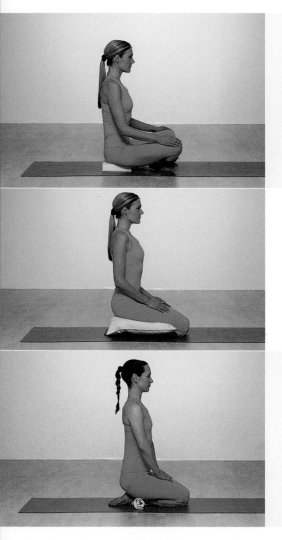

FOAM BLOCK

A firm foam block will help if your hips are stiff or you find it difficult to lengthen the spine in sitting postures, because it optimizes the tilt of the pelvis. If your neck is uncomfortable when you are lying on your back, you may find it useful to have a block as a support under your head.

PILLOW

A pillow can be used instead of a block to sit on or to rest your head on. It can also be used as a support to help relieve muscular tension. When kneeling, a pillow can be placed under the bent knees to help relieve tension in the inner thigh muscles.

ROLLED TOWEL

Kneeling positions can put strain on stiff ankles. To relieve this, roll up a towel firmly and place it between the ankles and the floor. A folded towel can also be used under bony parts of the feet or ankles, especially if you are working on a hard floor.

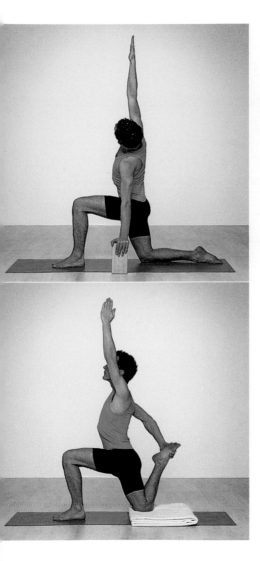

WOODEN BLOCK

Blocks can be used in a wide variety of situations as supports and stabilizers to help you practice postures effectively without straining yourself. If using a block in the Chandra sequence (see left and p.83) or in Triangle (see p.38), consider the block as an extension of your arm, and position it carefully so that your final posture maintains alignment. Check the placing of the block before you move into your posture.

FOLDED BLANKET

A blanket can be used for support in sitting, kneeling, and inverted postures, and to keep warm in relaxation and meditation. In a state of deep relaxation, the body temperature can drop considerably, so it is wise to cover up with a blanket before you start practicing your relaxation technique.

basic
breathing

There is a fundamental connection between the breath and your physical, mental, and emotional states. In yoga, the breath is how vital energy – "the breath behind the breath" – enters the body.

Breathing well is of fundamental importance for health. Breathing provides oxygen for the metabolic processes from which we derive the energy to move, think, and feel, and carries away carbon dioxide, the main waste product of metabolism. Physical tension in the respiratory muscles between the ribs can cause tightness in the chest, and even chest pain. Relaxed breathing techniques will release tension from the whole of the upper body, improving your ability to adjust your breathing to meet changing requirements.

The breath also provides a powerful link between mind and body. By controlling your breathing patterns – for example, the rhythm and depth of breathing, the length of the out-breath, and the balance between right and left nostrils – you can influence your physical, mental, and emotional states.

Good breathing habits

Yoga encourages breathing through the nose, full use of the diaphragm, a slow, smooth breathing pattern, and coordination of movement and breath. Opening movements, such as back bends, are practiced on the in-breath, and closing movements, such as forward bends, on the out-breath.

Full Yogic Breath (see opposite) helps develop awareness of the action of respiratory muscles and encourages good breathing habits. It is essential to building self-esteem, and can be done lying down, standing, or sitting.

full yogic breath

This breathing practice induces calm, harmonizing breath and body. After completing Step 3, combine all three steps to produce full, continuous in- and out-breaths. This is called the complete breath. Do five rounds.

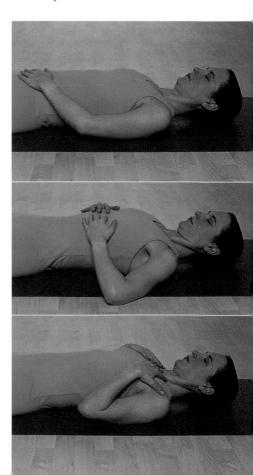

1 Lie on your back with your palms resting on your abdomen, the middle fingers just touching. Breathe into your hands, feeling the abdomen swell out and the fingers move apart as you breathe in. Then feel the abdomen sink back as you exhale. Repeat three times. This is abdominal breathing.

2 Bring your hands to your ribcage, with your fingers to the front and thumbs on the back ribs. On the in-breath, feel the ribs expand into the hands as the chest swells out. As you exhale, let the chest deflate and the hands sink down. Repeat three times like this.

3 Place your fingers on your collarbones, in front of your shoulders. Breathe in, and feel the the top of the chest expand and the fingers rise up toward the head. As you breathe out, feel the chest and fingers sink back down. Repeat three times like this.

breath with
movement

These simple postures are designed to deepen your connection with your breath, as well as gently moving the joints. Each movement is timed to match the length of the breath.

arm stretch 1

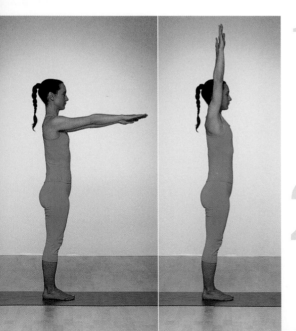

1 Practice the complete breath (see p.23) five times. Then, on an inhalation, raise the arms in front of you to shoulder height. Have the wrists, elbows, and shoulders in line, and the arms shoulder-width apart. Exhale.

2 On the next inhalation, extend the arms up directly above the head. Imagine a vertical line from your fingers to your ankles, aligning wrists, ears, and shoulders. Exhaling, return the arms to horizontal. Repeat the movement five times.

arm stretch 2

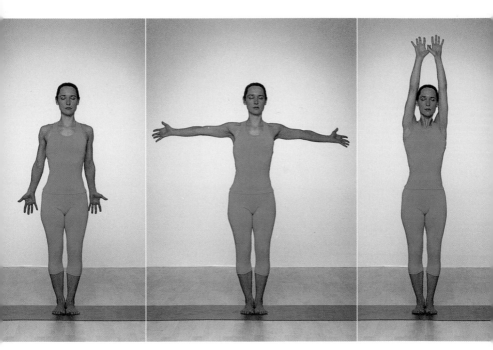

1 Stand with your feet together. As you exhale, turn the palms to face the front and pull the arms back, drawing the shoulder blades toward each other behind. Take a complete breath.

2 Starting to inhale, raise the arms up to shoulder height and out to the sides, extending the stretch right up to the fingertips. Keep the palms of the hands facing forward.

3 Still inhaling, extend the arms above your head, keeping them behind your ears. Feel the chest open. Exhale, lowering the arms by the sides, palms facing the front. Repeat the movement five times.

arm stretch 3

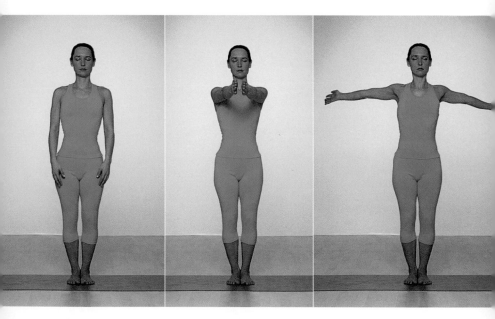

Stand up straight, feet together. Close your eyes. On an out-breath, release the shoulders down away from the ears. Let the palms rest on the thighs. Take a complete breath (see p.23), feeling it move through the body.

On an inhalation, let the arms float up to shoulder height. Turn the hands so the palms are facing each other and bring them close enough together to be able to feel the heat from each palm without the hands touching. Exhale.

As you inhale, open the arms out wide to the sides. Keep moving the arms back until you complete your inhalation with a fully open chest. Return to Step 2 as you exhale. Repeat Steps 2 and 3 seven times with your eyes closed.

energy-releasing pose

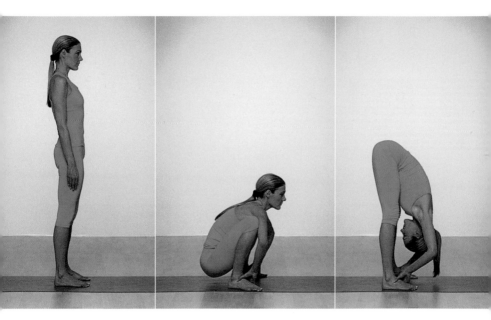

1 This practice develops synchronization between breath and movement, releasing energy and building strength. Stand with your feet hip-width apart, toes pointing forward, arms by your side. Look straight ahead and breathe in.

2 As you exhale, bend your knees and squat, tucking your fingers under the instep of each foot. Inhale, lengthening the spine and neck to look up. Point the elbows out and keep the tops of your thighs close to the lower belly.

3 As you exhale, straighten your legs, lifting your bottom toward the ceiling. Let your head hang down low so you can look between your calves. Keep the hands under the feet. Repeat Steps 2 and 3 five to seven times.

elbow circling

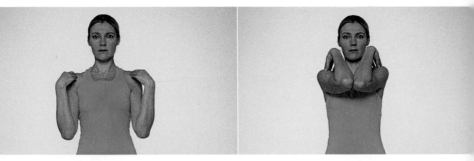

1 Breathing in, stretch out the arms in front of you. Turn the palms up, bend the elbows, and rest the fingers on the shoulders. Breathing out, let the elbows drop down to the waist.

2 On the next in-breath, lift the elbows out in front of your body at shoulder height, keeping the fingers on the shoulders. Pull the elbows toward each other until they touch.

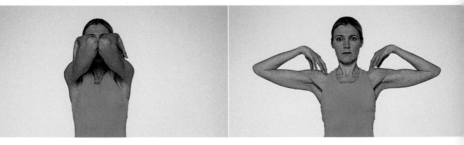

3 Still breathing in, lift the elbows higher in front of you, pointing them up toward the ceiling. Make sure the elbows do not separate.

4 As you breathe out, let the elbows separate and move the arms out at shoulder height. Roll the elbows back and down in a circular motion. Repeat Steps 2 to 4 three to seven times.

yogic rock and roll

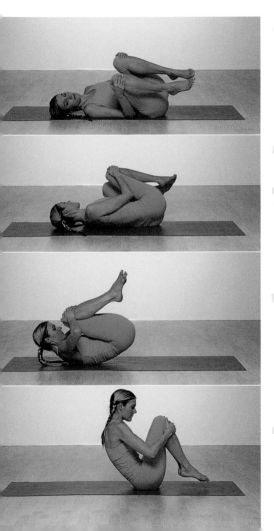

1 Lie on your back and take a complete breath (see p.23). On an in-breath, bend the knees and bring them up on each side of the abdomen. Hold a knee with each hand and rock to one side.

2 Breathing out, roll your body over to the other side. Roll from side to side like this several times. Then center your body.

3 As you breathe in, rock back gently along the length of the spine. Keep your back rounded and your legs tucked on each side of your abdomen.

4 As you breathe out, rock forward along the length of the spine. Rock back and forth like this several times. Finally, on an out-breath, come up to sitting.

pulling the rope

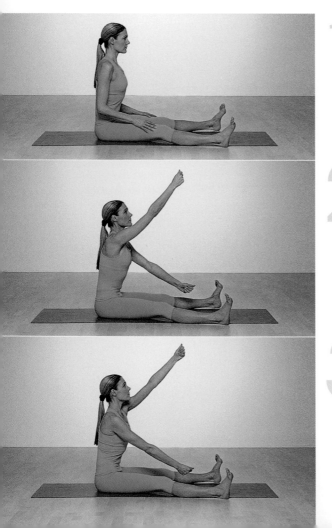

1 Sit with the legs straight out in front a little over hip-width apart. Keep the spine straight and lift up from the hips. Place your hands just above your knees. Flex your feet. Look straight ahead.

2 On an inhalation, reach your right hand up as high as it will go, and a little in front, as if to grab hold of an imaginary bell rope. Keep the arm straight and look up at the hand. Straighten and lift the left arm as if to hold the rope lower down.

3 On an exhalation, move the right hand down as if pulling the rope. Keep a stretch right through to the hand and move the trunk forward from the hips. Repeat Steps 2 and 3 on the left side. Then alternate right and left five to seven times.

rowing the boat

1 Sit with legs together, straight out in front. Push the heels away and lift up from the hips. Take an abdominal breath. Hold the arms out in front at shoulder level and make two fists as if holding the handles of a pair of oars. Exhale.

2 On an inhalation, lean back as far as you find comfortable, pulling the imaginary pair of oars. Bend the elbows and tuck them down into the waist. Feel the stretch in the abdomen.

3 On an exhalation, move the body forward as far as you can, reaching the arms straight out over the toes. Feel the stretch in the lower back. Repeat Steps 2 and 3 five to seven times, moving with the breath.

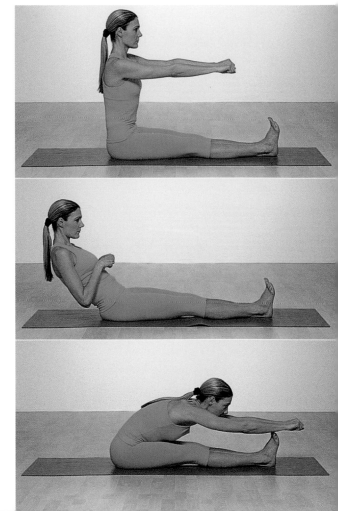

stirring the pot

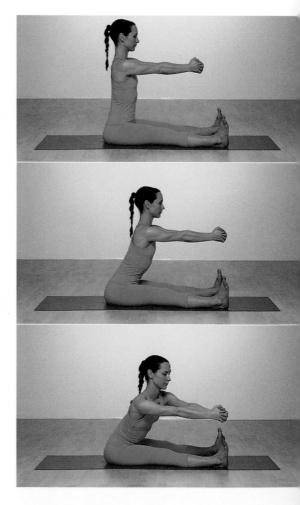

1 Sit up straight, your legs in front as far apart as is comfortable. Sit forward on your sitting bones and extend your arms straight out in front, at shoulder height. Interlock your fingers so the right thumb is on top.

2 Imagine that you are holding a huge wooden spoon and that there is an enormous pot of oatmeal placed between your heels. Exhale as you move forward from the hips, keeping your arms at shoulder height.

3 Still exhaling, move your body and arms over your right foot. This is the beginning of a circular motion as you stir the imaginary pot of oatmeal between your heels.

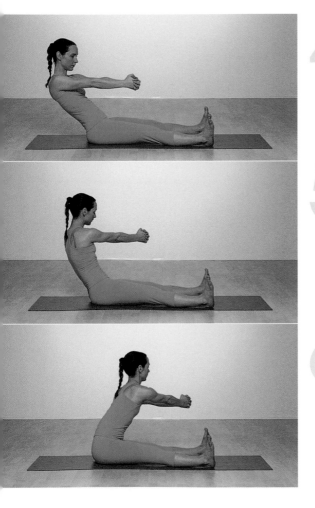

Continue in a clockwise direction. Inhale as you lean back, still moving from the hips, until your hands are positioned over your right thigh.

Still leaning back and breathing in, move your body to the left, bringing your hands over your left thigh. Feel the stretch in the pelvis and abdomen.

Breathing out, move your body forward so your hands are over your left foot. This completes one circle. Repeat the circular motion 10 times clockwise. Pause, resting your arms, and repeat 10 times, with the left thumb on top, in a counter-clockwise direction.

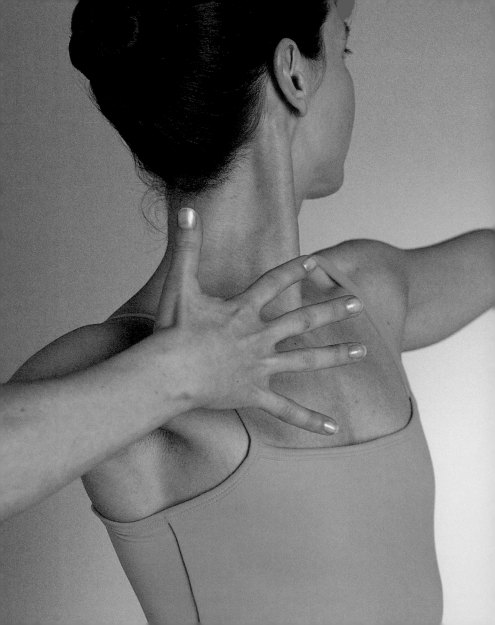

building
blocks

This section presents a variety of postures and other yoga practices to promote awareness and develop self-confidence. Stay in the postures only for as long as you are able to hold them steadily and comfortably, breathing evenly. Listen to your body as you practice.

bow and
arrow

Promoting balanced strength, clear focus, and an open heart, this posture works deep into the muscles around the neck and shoulder blades to release tension and relieve stiffness and cramp.

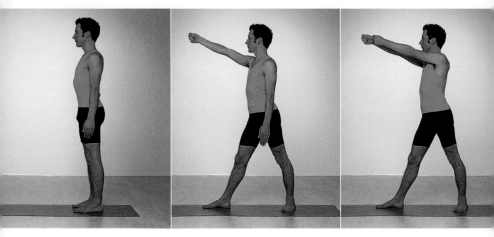

1 Stand with your feet shoulder-width apart, arms by your sides. Step the right foot forward 2 ft (60 cm). Turn the left foot out 45 degrees.

2 Clench your right hand and, inhaling, raise your right arm up and out above shoulder level, over the right foot. Gaze at the right thumb.

3 Tuck the thumb of the left hand into the palm and wrap the fingers around it. Exhaling, raise the left arm to bring the left hand up against the inside of the right wrist.

4 On the next inhalation, slowly bend the left elbow as you draw the left hand back to your chin and then behind the left ear, as though drawing on a bow. Tense the muscles in both arms. Exhale, and then take a breath in.

5 Exhale as you open the fingers of the left hand, as though releasing an imaginary arrow from the bow. Still exhaling, relax the neck and bring the left fist forward to bring the left hand level with the right hand. Then, draw back the bow on an in-breath and release on an out-breath five times. On the next out-breath, lower both arms to your sides. Then repeat the entire sequence on the other side.

Focus on thumb

Elbow and shoulder in line

Lifting up from lower back

Keep legs straight and heels grounded

triangle

Triangle builds physical strength, lifts the spirits, improves emotional confidence, and promotes balance. It stretches spine and abdomen, strengthens legs and feet, and promotes flexibility in the hips.

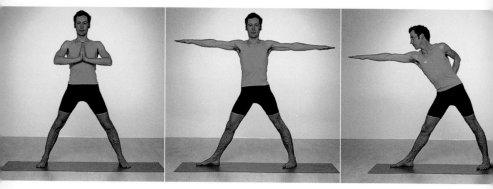

1 Stand with your feet about 3 ft (1 m) apart and bring your palms together in front of your chest. Exhale.

2 As you breathe in, sweep your arms out to the side at shoulder height. Turn your right foot so the toes point to the side. Turn your left heel out.

3 As you exhale, reach out with the right arm, extending it as far as it will go. Bend the left arm and rest the palm of the hand in the small of the back.

TAKE CARE
• If you have back problems, rest front arm higher up the leg.
• Do not turn your head to look up at your hand if you have neck problems.

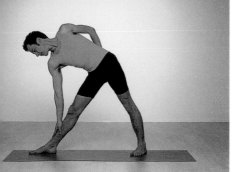

Still breathing out, lower the right arm to rest on the thigh and then slide it down the right leg. Keep the weight on the outside edges of your feet. Look at your right foot.

Make a straight line with arms

Keep upper body lifted, chest open

On an in-breath, extend your left arm straight up above your head, pointing the fingers toward the ceiling. Turn your head to look up at the left hand. To come out of the pose, on an in-breath, move your body back into an upright position, allowing the arms to move back to the horizontal. Turn your feet to face forward. Bring your palms together in front of your chest. Take a complete breath, then repeat the sequence on the other side.

Press outside edge of foot to floor

tree

An elegant balance, this posture promotes concentration and develops strength in the legs and feet. Coordinating the quietening of mind and body, Tree pose is an effective antidote to anxiety.

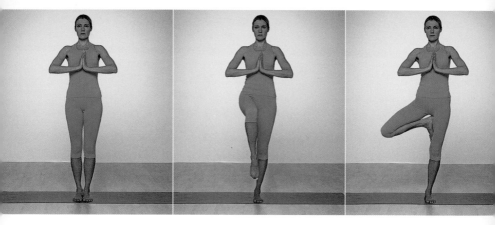

1 Stand with your legs and feet together. Bring your arms in front of your chest and push the heels of your hands firmly together, thumbs against chest. Inhale.

2 Exhale as you sink your weight into the left foot. On the next in-breath, raise the right knee up in front of you as high as it will comfortably go.

3 Turn the right knee out to the right side, and bring the sole of the right foot onto the inside of the left thigh. Keep your palms together. Take a complete breath.

Point fingers
toward ceiling

Keep your
eyes focused
at a point at
eye level

Make sure
fronts of both
hips face
directly
forward

If you feel balanced, on the next
inhalation, raise the hands up above
the head, keeping the palms together,
and holding your focus on a point
straight ahead. Take a complete
breath. To come out of the pose, on
an exhalation, bring the arms back
down to your sides and lower your
right foot to the floor. Take a few
rounds of breath, then repeat the
pose on the other side.

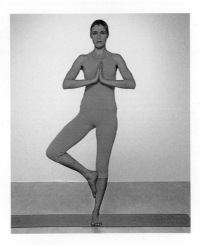

ALTERNATIVE

If you find it difficult to balance in the full
pose, try bringing the sole of your right
foot to rest just below the knee. If you
have HBP, do not raise your arms above
your head. Avoid the pose if you have
arthritis in the knees or back problems.

dancer

This strong and energizing practice opens the chest and promotes excellent coordination and balance. The pose of the Dancer develops focus together with strength of mind and body.

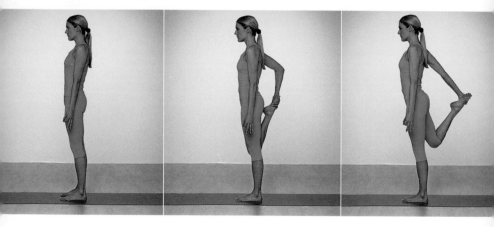

1 Stand with your legs together, arms by your sides. Look straight ahead. Press the tip of the left thumb against the tip of the left index finger, to make a circle. Exhale.

2 Bend the right knee and take the right foot behind you, catching hold of it with your right hand. Hold the foot close to the right buttock. Take a breath in.

3 On the next out-breath, slowly raise the right knee behind you to a comfortable height, still holding the foot. Keep your balance steady and your eyes focused.

Lengthen spine

4 On the next in-breath, raise the left hand to at least chin height. Focus the gaze on the hand. Breathe fully and easily for three rounds. To come out of the pose, on an out-breath, lower your left arm to your side, release your right foot, and lower the knee, and then the foot. Repeat on the other side.

Move knee up and back

Keep left leg straight

TAKE CARE
• Be careful not to collapse the back in the full pose: keep the back lengthened.
• Raise the knee behind you only as high as is comfortable.

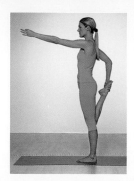

ALTERNATIVE
If you find it difficult to raise the knee behind you in the full pose without losing balance, practice with the knees side-by-side. Work slowly to bring the heel close to the buttock, feeling the stretch in the thigh.

boat

An instant energizer that builds strength, promotes confidence, and develops concentration, Boat pose strengthens abdominal, back, and leg muscles, boosts circulation, and helps eliminate anxiety.

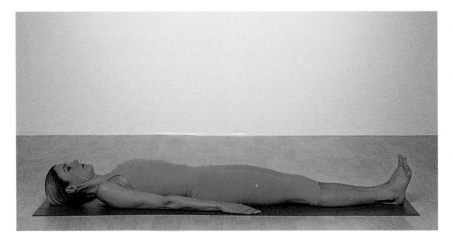

TAKE CARE
Avoid this practice if you have HBP, a heart condition, slipped disk, or sciatica.

1 Lie on your back, with your arms by your sides, shoulders well away from your ears, and palms down. Have your legs straight and together. Observe the rise and fall of the abdominal breath (see p.23).

2 Keeping your focus on the abdomen, take a deep breath in and hold it inside as you raise your arms, shoulders, head, trunk, and legs up about 4 in (10 cm) off the ground. Keeping your arms and legs straight, extend your hands toward the toes, and draw the toes in toward your head. Keep the hands and feet at roughly the same height as you balance on your buttocks.

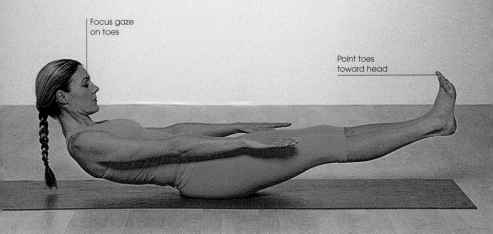

Focus gaze
on toes

Point toes
toward head

3 When you are ready to exhale, slowly lower the legs, trunk, and head back onto the floor. Rest with arms and legs by your sides to release all body tension. Repeat three to five times.

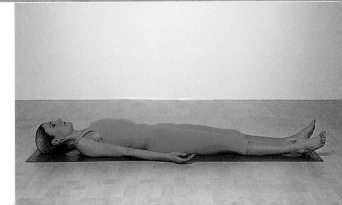

downward
dog

An invigorating stretch, Downward Dog strengthens the limbs and relieves tightness in the back and shoulders. This classic inversion is a powerful energy booster.

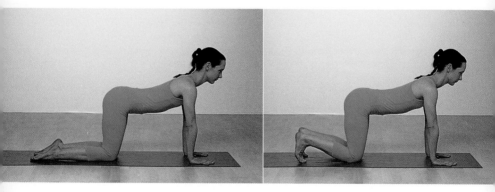

1 Begin on all fours, the hands directly under the shoulders, the feet and knees hip-width apart. Look slightly ahead. Take a breath in.

2 Maintaining the position of your hands and knees, lift your feet and tuck your toes under. Continue to look at the floor slightly ahead.

TAKE CARE
• If you have a back problem, do the posture cautiously with your knees bent throughout.
• If you have HBP, a heart condition, glaucoma, or a detached retina, do the posture with your hands on a chair.

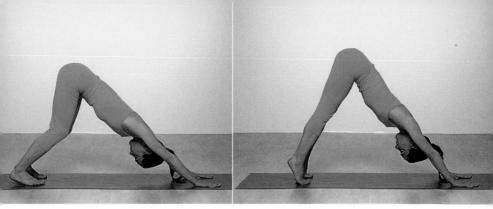

3 On an out-breath, lift your hips up and back. Keeping your knees bent, push your hands against the floor to send your weight back toward your feet. Lengthen through the spine. Let your head hang between your arms.

4 Straighten your legs, coming up onto your toes as you lift your sitting bones up to the ceiling. Lengthen through your back and keep your neck relaxed and your head hanging. Take a breath in.

Lengthen through backs of legs

Bring heels as near to floor as possible

5 On an out-breath, bring your heels toward the floor as you lengthen through the backs of the legs. Breathe evenly in the posture, then lower the knees to the floor and return to the starting position on an out-breath,

Head relaxed between arms

lunge
warrior

A powerful and poised practice, Lunge Warrior promotes flexibility
the hips and opens the hips and thighs. It also encourages steady
focus and stability of balance.

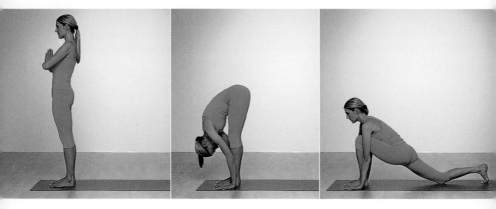

1 Stand up straight, feet
together, arms by your
side. Bring your palms
together in front of
your chest.

2 As you breathe
out, fold your body
forward from the hips,
bending the knees
slightly. Place your
palms on the floor on
each side of your feet.
Take a breath in.

3 As you breathe out,
bend the knees, and
take a large step back
with your right foot.
Land on the ball of
the right foot. Rest
your upper body on
your left thigh. Look
slightly ahead.

Look
ahead

As you breathe in, extend the right heel backward, and for a stronger stretch, bring the knee off the floor. Lengthen through the upper body and look straight ahead. Breathe steadily. Step the right foot forward, come back up to standing, and repeat on the other side.

Knee in
line with
ankle

Heel pushes
backward

ALTERNATIVE

If you have back problems, HBP, or a heart condition, do not lift your right knee off the ground in the full pose. Allow the weight of the hips to sink down and through into the grounded knee.

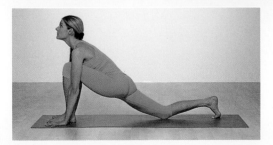

cobra

Cobra extends the spine, strengthening the back muscles and opening the chest. It is a valuable posture for developing a sense of power and grace, boosting self-confidence.

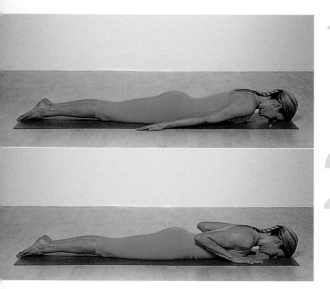

1 Lie on your front, forehead on the floor and feet together with heels touching. Let your arms lie down by your sides, palms facing down. Exhale.

2 Place your hands under the shoulders, spread your fingers, middle finger pointing forward. Keep the elbows close to the body and tuck your tailbone under.

TAKE CARE
• Avoid if you have facet joint problems in the spine.
• If you have arthritis in the neck, keep the head in line with the spine.

3 As you breathe in, slide the forehead forward to lift the forehead, nose, chin, and then the shoulders and chest. Use the back muscles to lift the upper body off the floor. Focus on taking the chest forward, lengthening through the front of the body and extending throughout the spine. Breathe easily. There should be no feeling of strain.

Extend spine

Relax shoulders

4 Repeat the pose once or twice, then relax for a few minutes. Bring your arms forward, and fold one under the other. Turn your head to one side and rest your face on your forearms. Close your eyes.

snake

This backward bend stretches the front of the body, opens the chest, and promotes easeful movement in the upper back. Taking the arms back helps relieve stiffness in the shoulders and the mid-back.

1 Lie flat on your front with your forehead on the floor and your arms by your sides, palms face down. Have your legs straight, your heels together. Exhale.

2 Breathing in, lift your arms up and bring them behind your back. Move your elbows as close together as you can. Place the palms of your hands together and interlock the fingers. Roll your shoulders down and back away from your ears, squeezing your shoulder blades together. Exhale.

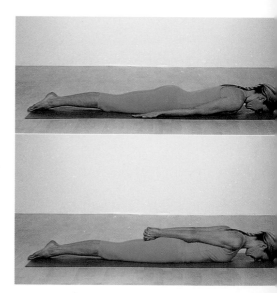

TAKE CARE
Do not practice this posture if you have a peptic ulcer or a hernia.

As you breathe in, lift your head and raise the front of your chest up away from the floor. Look straight ahead. Exhale.

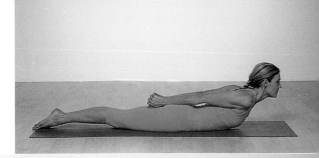

On the next inhalation, lift the arms up away from the back and move your hands away toward your feet. Keep the arms and hands together. Hold the posture for up to seven complete breaths. Feel your abdomen moving against the floor as you breathe.

Keep neck long and shoulders well away from ears

Squeeze shoulder blades together

Keep heels pressing together

On an exhalation, slowly lower the arms back down onto the back, tuck in the chin, and rest the forehead on the floor.

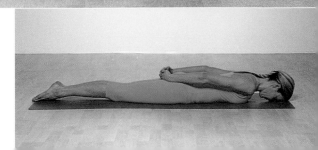

resting
crocodile

Resting Crocodile is a healing posture for many types of back pain, including slipped disk, sciatica, and lower back pain. It also encourages full and complete breathing.

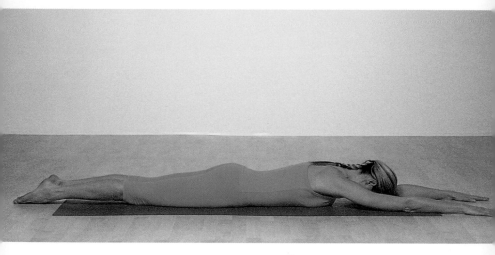

TAKE CARE
• Let your feet and ankles relax. Point toes in toward each other or out to the sides.
• Feel the abdomen moving against the floor as you inhale.

1 Lie flat on your front, your feet hip-width apart and your arms outstretched above your head. Rest your forehead on the floor. This is known as the Reverse Corpse pose.

2 On an in-breath, bend your elbows, and bring the heels of your hands together. Raise your head and shoulders, and rest your chin in the palms of your hands. Stay in the posture for several breaths.

Gaze straight ahead

Upper back at a comfortable angle

Legs and buttocks relaxed

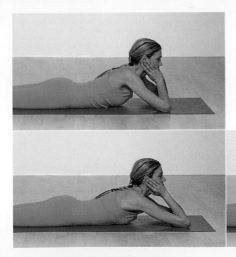

ALTERNATIVES

Take your elbows wider apart to spread the upper back and neck. Move your elbows farther in front to lessen the angle of the curve in your back. Bring the elbows closer to the body to increase the angle of the curve in your back.

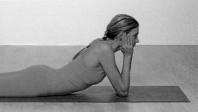

sun salute

The Sun Salute synchronizes breath with movement and promoting fluidity, endurance, strength, and adaptability. Best practiced early in the day, it harmonizes and energizes the whole body system.

1 Stand tall, with feet together and chest lifted. Inhale. On the out-breath, bring the palms of the hands together in the center of the chest in prayer position. Breathe into the heart space.

2 On the next in-breath, lift your hands over the head, straightening the arms, and turn the palms to face the sun in front of you. Lean back a little. Open the heart with your in-breath to feel strong and confident.

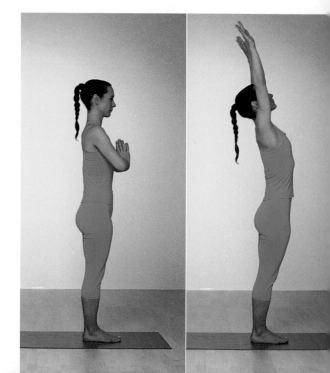

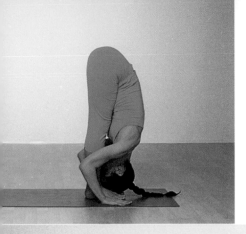

3 Exhaling, bend forward from the hips into a Forward Bend. Keep a long spine and bend your knees if you need to. Maintain a sense of one continuous line from the bottom of your spine to the tips of your fingers. Bring the hands flat on the floor on each side of your feet, fingers pointing forward. Tuck your head into your shins. Be soft.

4 On the next in-breath, keeping your palms flat on the floor, step your right leg as far back as you can into Lunge Warrior (see p.48). Let the right knee bend and rest on the floor. Keep the toes tucked under. If you need to, steeple the fingers. Bring your chest forward and draw your focus up to the point between your eyebrows as you raise your face up to soak up the energizing rays of the sun. ▶

Tuck toes under

Allow knee to touch floor

Keep left knee directly above ankle

5 On the next exhalation, bring your left foot back to join your right, straighten your knees, and swing your tailbone up high. Straighten your arms and lift your shoulders back away from your ears. Lift up on your toes, and then lengthen through the backs of the legs to bring the heels down toward the floor into Downward Dog (see p.46).

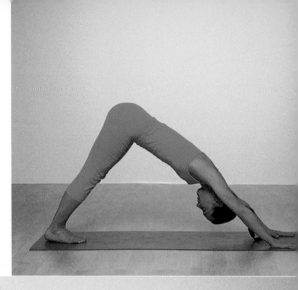

6 Let there be a pause in the breath as you lower your chest to the floor. Lower the head so that the nose touches the floor, too. Keep your bottom in the air and bend your knees until they touch the floor. Focus your attention on your abdomen.

Lift buttocks
toward
ceiling

Lower chest to
floor directly
between hands

7 As you inhale, bring your abdomen to the floor and raise the upper chest away from the floor to come into Cobra (see p.50). Lengthen through the spine and neck. Feel a firm contact between the pubic bone and the floor. Look ahead.

Tuck elbows in close to your sides

8 On the next exhalation, come into Downward Dog again. Tuck your toes under, straighten your knees, and swing your tailbone up high. Straighten your arms and move your shoulders back away from your ears. Lift up on your toes, and then lengthen through the backs of the legs to bring the heels down toward the floor. Let your head hang down between your arms. Relax the neck. ►

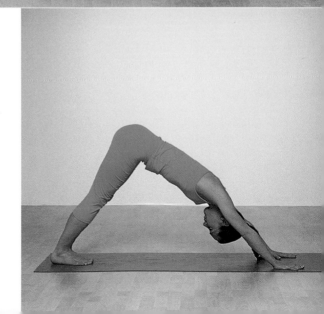

On the next inhalation, bring your right knee forward and come into Lunge Warrior again. Put the sole of the right foot flat on the ground next to the thumb of your right hand. Have the tops of the toes and fingers level. Bring your chest forward and draw your focus up to the point between your eyebrows as you raise up your face to soak up the energizing rays of the sun.

Lengthen spine

Keep knee in line with ankle

Keep toes tucked under

10 On the next exhalation, come back into a Forward Bend, bringing your left foot forward to join your right. Keep your hands flat on the floor, fingers pointing forward, and bend your knees if you need to. Have your head tucked into your shins and keep the focus of your attention at the base of your spine. Be soft, accepting of where you are able to be in the pose.

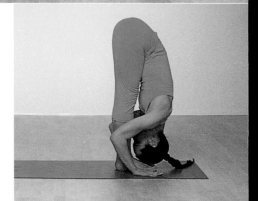

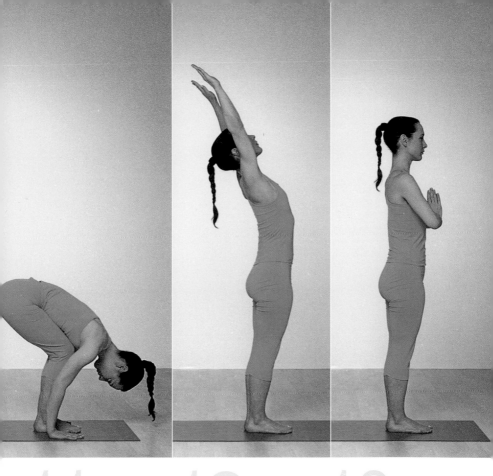

On the next in-breath, bend your knees and start to lift your body back up to standing, pivoting from the hips and keeping neck in line with spine.

Continuing to breathe in, bring your arms up above your head. Keeping the arms straight and long, lean back a little and open your heart to feel strong and confident.

On the next in-breath, bring the palms together above the head. Breathing out, lower them until they come to the center of the chest. Breathe into the heart space.

thunderbolt

This useful meditation posture aligns the spine, neck, and head, and promotes flexibility in the ankles and feet. The quiet that it brings to the body is conducive to digestion.

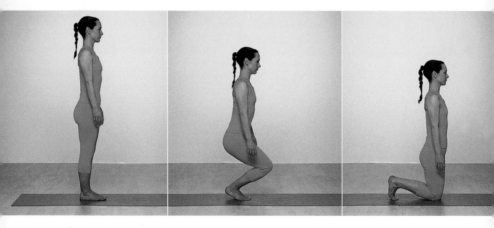

1 Stand with your feet together and arms by your sides. Look straight ahead. Inhale.

2 As you exhale, keeping your knees together, lower them forward and down to the floor.

3 With your thighs vertical, bring the big toes together and the heels apart. Untuck the toes so the tops of the feet are on the floor. Keep the spine straight. Inhale.

As you exhale, lower the buttocks onto the feet, and let your heels touch the sides of your hips. Place your hands just above your knees, palms down. Breathe evenly for a few minutes. To come out of the posture, tuck the toes under and lift the knees up off the floor. On an inhalation, return to standing.

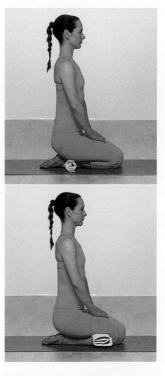

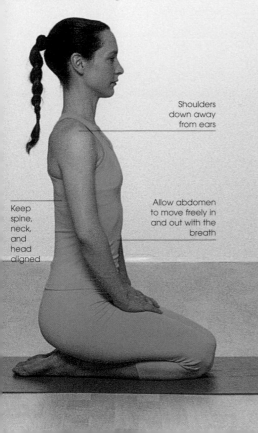

Shoulders down away from ears

Keep spine, neck, and head aligned

Allow abdomen to move freely in and out with the breath

ALTERNATIVES

If you find that your ankles ache, tuck a rolled blanket in the front of the ankle joint, between ankle and floor. If you have varicose veins or knee problems, try tucking a rolled blanket between your knees and your calves. If you feel any discomfort in the thighs, separate the knees slightly.

philosopher

A rapid route to physical and mental relaxation, this pose develops the powers of concentration and enables clarity of thought. It encourages a quiet, contemplative self-confidence.

1 Start by kneeling in Thunderbolt pose (see p.62) with your knees together and the palms of your hands resting on your thighs. Sit back on your heels and straighten your spine. Look straight ahead. Take a complete breath. As you exhale, settle your weight down. Let your awareness travel within.

TAKE CARE
Keep the spine and neck extended, feeling a continuous line from the tailbone to the top of the head.

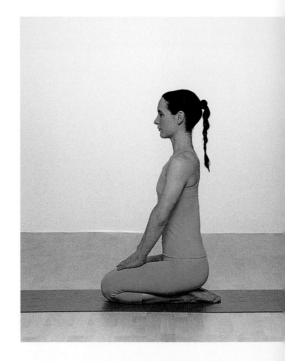

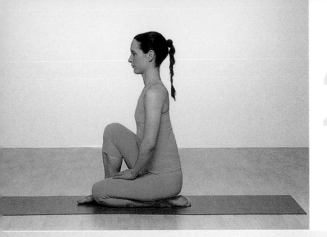

2 Inhale as you lift up the right knee, and put the sole of the right foot flat on the floor to the inside of the left knee, bringing the right ankle directly underneath the right knee.

3 Exhaling, raise your right elbow and place it on top of the right knee. Rest your chin on the palm of the right hand. Close your eyes and focus on your breathing for two minutes, imagining that the breath is flowing in and out through a point between your eyebrows. To come out of the pose, lower the right hand and your right knee, and repeat on the left side.

Keep spine long, and head and neck aligned with spine

Ankle in line with knee

roaring lion

A potent antidote to introversion, this pose promotes a beautiful voice and gives you the confidence to use it. It stretches the face, jaw, and throat, and releases tension in the chest.

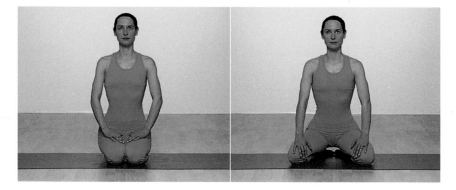

1 Kneel in Thunderbolt (see p.62) with your knees together and the palms of your hands on your thighs. If possible, face the sun. Inhale.

2 Exhale as you move your knees about 18 in (45 cm) apart. Spread out your fingers just above your knees, keeping your thumbs closest to your body.

TAKE CARE
• When you are comfortable with the practice, you may do up to 20 repetitions.
• If you have knee problems or painful wrists, sit on a chair. Lean forward, the hands placed lightly on the thighs.

Place your palms flat on the floor in between your knees with your fingers pointing back toward your body. Inhale. Lower your shoulders and keep your spine long and straight as you lean forward slightly. Exhale.

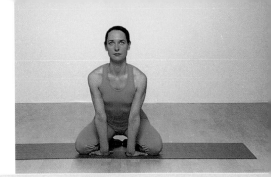

Push the chest forward as you inhale deeply through the nose. At the end of the inhalation, open your mouth as wide as possible and stick out your tongue, stretching the tip down toward your chin. On the exhalation, emit a long, breathy "aaaahhh" sound, like a soft roar, from the back of your throat. Feel the sound and the breath pouring out along the tongue. At the end of the "aaaahhh," put your tongue back inside the mouth and close the lips. Repeat the roar between three and seven times.

Keep neck long and chin lifted up high, so front of throat is stretched

When you have completed your chosen number of rounds, release the hands and, on an exhalation, fold forward from the hips to bring your forehead to the floor and arms beside your body. Stay for several breaths.

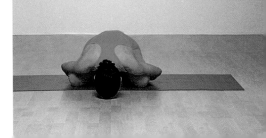

camel

Energizing and revitalizing, this powerful backward bend requires and promotes confidence and trust. It stretches the front of the body and opens the chest, relieving tension in the upper back.

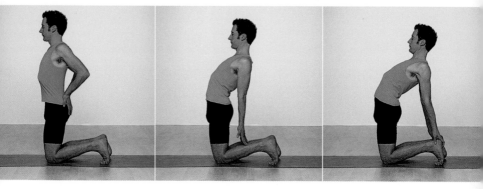

1 Kneel with knees hip-width apart. Tuck the toes under. Place your palms on the buttocks. Breathe in.

2 Keeping the spine extended, slowly move the hands down your thighs until they reach the shins.

3 Push the chest forward with an out-breath and grasp the heels. Draw the shoulder blades together behind you, opening the chest.

TAKE CARE

• If you have HBP, heart disease, back problems, hernia, or have had recent abdominal surgery, do not go beyond Step 2.

• If you have neck problems, do not take head back at Step 4.

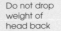

When you feel balanced, with your weight shared evenly between the knees and hands, point the chin up to the ceiling, keeping the back of the neck long. Stay in the pose for three breaths. To come out of the pose, slowly move the chin down and the hands back up the legs to the buttocks. On an inhalation, release the hands and return to the vertical position.

Do not drop weight of head back

Keep chest and abdomen moving rhythmically while breathing easily

Shoulders down from ears and spine extended

Thighs as vertical as possible

On an exhalation, fold forward into Child (see p.72) and lengthen the spine. Breathe into the abdomen and feel it moving against the thighs. Rest in this pose for a few minutes.

cat

Synchronizing breath and movement, Cat pose creates a strong link between mind and body. It eases tension in the spine and develops a full and effective yogic breath (see p.23).

1 Start in the all-fours position, with the palms flat on the floor directly under the shoulders, and the fingers well spread and pointing forward. Push the hands into the floor to prevent the shoulders from sagging. Look down at the floor. Take an in-breath.

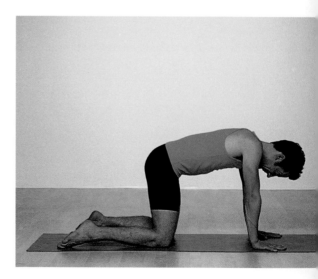

TAKE CARE
If you have weak wrists, support the body by placing one or both forearms on a pile of blocks or books.

2 On an exhalation, tuck your chin down into your chest, tuck in your tailbone, and suck your abdomen into your spine. The back should be rounded right over. Press the heels of the hands down into the floor and open up a space between the shoulder blades.

Round lower back

Keep back of neck long

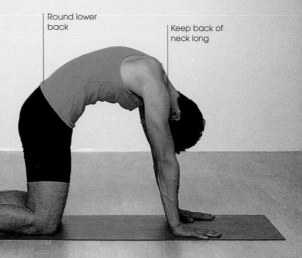

3 As you inhale, begin to lift the tailbone up away from the floor, so that the lower back dips toward the floor. Continue to lift the tailbone and feel first the middle of the back dip, then the upper back. Look at the floor in front of you. Alternate Steps 2 and 3 several times, feeling the movement spread from the base of the spine to the neck. Exhale and come into Hare (see p.74).

Allow abdomen to move down and lower back to dip a little

Look forward with a soft throat

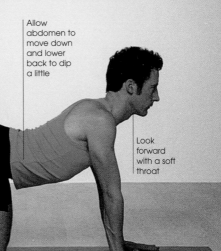

child

Quietening and calming, Child pose provides a long stretch through the spine, and easeful rest for shoulders and neck. It is excellent for developing awareness of the abdominal breath (see p.23).

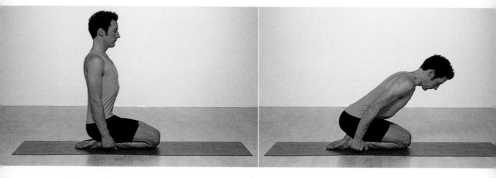

1 Kneel and sit back on your heels. Let your arms hang down on each side of the body. Lengthen through the spine and look straight ahead. Breathe in.

2 As you breathe out, fold forward slowly from the hips. Keep your buttocks on your heels and your arms by your sides.

TAKE CARE
• If you cannot sit on your heels, place a pillow beneath the buttocks.
• If you find it difficult to bring your head to the floor, rest it on two fists, one on top of the other. • If you have HBP, a detached retina, glaucoma, or back problems, rest your head on the seat of a chair.

Continue to fold forward, tucking the chin in to bring the forehead to the floor. Allow the weight of the arms to pull the shoulders gently toward the floor. Stay for several breaths.

Rounded back opens space between shoulders

Neck soft with weight of head supported on floor

Tailbone sinks down on heels

To come out of the pose, on an in-breath, bring the palms of your hands to the floor and begin to push up slowly. Gradually come back up to kneeling, your arms by your side, back straight.

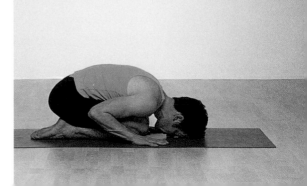

hare

This peaceful pose is soothing and quietening, providing relief from harsh self-criticism and anger. It also stretches the back and helps encourage good alignment of the spine.

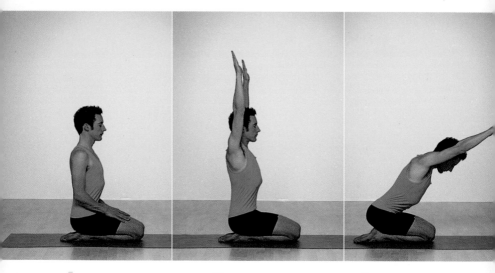

1 Sit in Thunderbolt pose (see p.62). Keep your back long and rest the palms of your hands on the thighs.

2 Inhale as you raise your arms above the head. Make a straight line from fingertips to the base of the spine.

3 Exhale as you fold forward from the hips, extending the fingertips forward as you come down.

Bring your forehead and the palms of your hands to rest on the floor at the same time. Extend the arms away in front of you, feeling an open space under your armpits. Breathe fully and easily in the pose. On an inhalation, keeping the head between the arms, and the back straight, return to a vertical position.

Allow upper back to open and relax

Extend arms forward

Sink weight of buttocks down onto heels

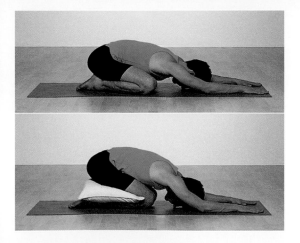

ALTERNATIVES

If you find it uncomfortable to keep your knees together, allow them to come a little apart. If you are not comfortable sitting back on your heels, place a pillow between your heels and your buttocks. If you have HBP, a detached retina, glaucoma, or back problems, stretch forward with your hands on the seat of a chair.

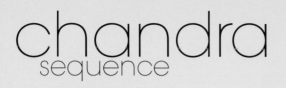

chandra
sequence

Requiring and promoting balance and strength, this sequence encourages fluidity of movement and sustained self-awareness. It energizes and releases the pelvic area.

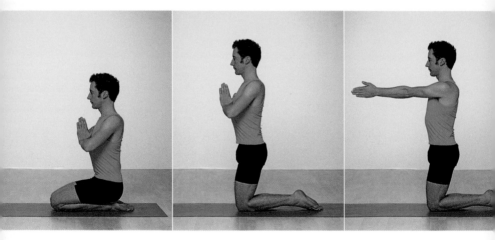

1 Start in Thunderbolt (see p.62). Bring the arms in front of your chest and press the heels of the hands together in prayer position. Exhale.

2 Inhale as you rise up onto the knees, keeping your back straight and your hands in front of you in prayer position.

3 As you breathe out, straighten your arms out in front of you, palms still pressed together, fingers pointing away from the body.

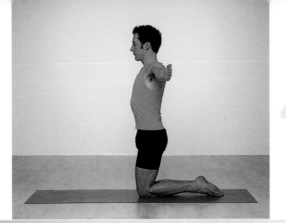

As you inhale, open your arms wide to the sides at shoulder height, keeping your arms straight.

Exhale as you step the left foot forward. Form a 90-degree angle, so the left knee is directly over the left ankle. Keep the arms spread wide. Take a breath in. ▶

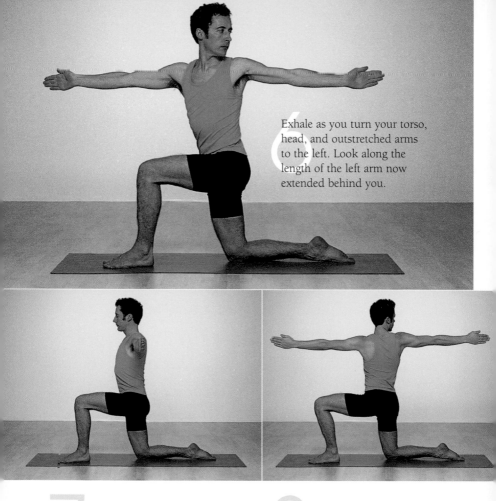

Exhale as you turn your torso, head, and outstretched arms to the left. Look along the length of the left arm now extended behind you.

Keeping both arms held out straight and at shoulder height, breathe in as you return to the front. Look directly in front of you.

Exhale as you turn your torso, head, and outstretched arms to the right. Look along the length of the right arm. Keep both arms straight and at shoulder height.

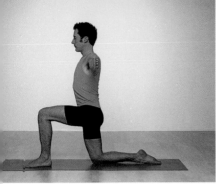

9 Keeping both arms straight and at shoulder height, inhale as you return to the front. Look directly in front of you.

10 Exhale as you bend at the waist to bring the left arm down to touch the floor with your fingertips. Stretch the right arm up, keeping a long straight line from the right fingertips to the left. Look up at the right hand. Take a breath in as you return to the center, keeping the arms wide.

11 Exhale as you bend at the waist to bring the right arm down to touch the floor with your fingertips. Stretch the left arm up, keeping a straight line from the left fingertips to the right. Look up at the left hand. Come back to Step 9 on the in-breath. ▶

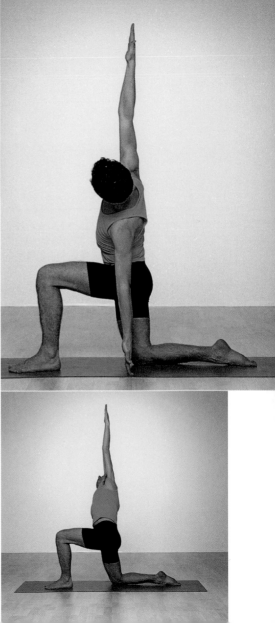

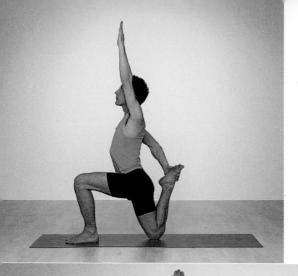

12

Exhale as you reach straight up with your left hand. At the same time, reach behind with your right hand to hold the toes of the right foot and pull the foot up toward the right buttock. Inhale as you extend the left hand up. Look up at the left hand. Release the right foot back to the floor and lower the left hand on an exhalation. Take a breath in.

13

Exhale as you reach straight up with your right hand. At the same time, reach behind you with your left hand to hold the toes of the right foot. Take a breath in as you extend the right hand up. Look up.

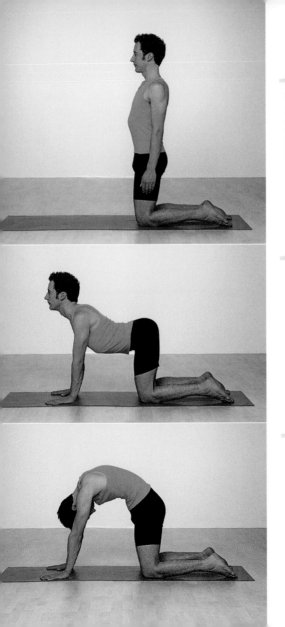

Release the right foot back to the floor and lower the right hand on an exhalation. Inhale. Exhale as you step your left foot back to return to Thunderbolt pose.

Bend at the waist to come down onto all fours. Have the palms flat on the floor directly under the shoulders, with the fingers spread and pointing forward. Inhale fully as you look forward and slightly up, lengthening through the whole spine as it dips slightly in Step 3 of Cat (see p.71).

On an exhalation, tuck your chin down into your chest, tuck in your tailbone, and suck your abdomen up to your spine in Step 2 of Cat. Press the heels of the hands down into the floor and open up a space between your shoulder blades. Inhale and look forward to come back to Step 15. ▶

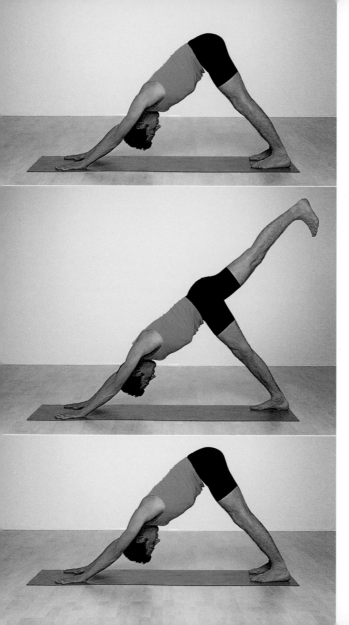

17 Exhale as you tuck your toes under and swing your tailbone up into Downward Dog (see p.46). Keep the elbows and knees strong and arms and legs straight.

18 Inhale as you raise the left leg up behind you, flexing the foot. Keep your neck relaxed and let your head hang between your arms.

19 Exhale as you place your left foot back on the floor, returning to Downward Dog. Take a full breath.

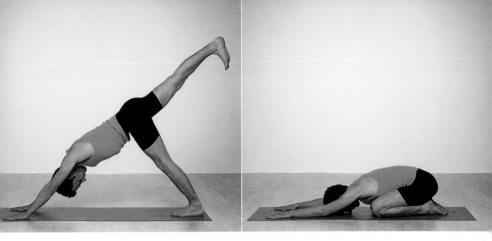

20 Inhale as you raise the right leg up behind you, flexing the foot. Exhale as you place your foot back on the floor. Breathe in.

21 Exhale as you bend your knees and lower your head to the floor, coming into Hare (see p.74). On an in-breath, come back up into Thunderbolt and repeat the sequence on the other side.

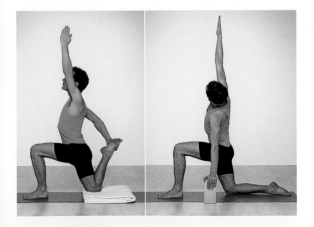

ALTERNATIVES
• If your knee feels uncomfortable in Steps 12 and 13, place a folded blanket beneath it. Have the blanket in place at the start of the sequence.
• If it is difficult to touch the floor in Steps 10 and 11 without losing balance, position a wooden block so you can rest the heel of your hand on it.

dolphin

The Dolphin pose is a vital part of the preparation for Headstand (see p.86). Until you can comfortably do 10 repetitions of this posture, you should not attempt to do Headstand.

1 Kneel on the floor with your hands resting lightly on your thighs and your buttocks resting on your heels. Inhale and then fold forward on an out-breath.

2 Inhale as you come onto your knees and elbows. Place your elbows under your shoulders and clasp each elbow with a hand.

3 Keeping the elbows still, slide your hands forward and interlock your fingers. Lift your shoulders back and down.

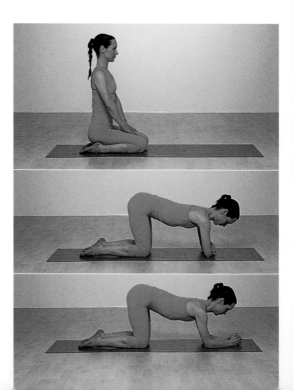

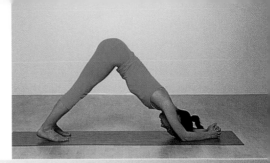

Breathing in, tuck your toes under and straighten your legs, so your buttocks lift and you feel the weight resting on your elbows and forearms. Keep your fingers interlocked.

Raise your head. As you breathe in, move your head and shoulders forward until the shoulders are over the hands. Feel the weight descending into your elbows and forearms. As you exhale, move back. If you can, repeat the move: inhale forward and exhale back. To come out of the pose, move back onto all fours, then bring your buttocks back onto the heels and rest in Hare (see p.74).

Keep head and neck parallel to floor as you move forward and backward

Keep shoulders down away from ears

TAKE CARE
• Avoid Dolphin if you have HBP, heart disease, glaucoma, or a detached retina.
• Avoid the pose if you are menstruating.

headstand

This is the "king" of all yoga postures, rejuvenating every system in the body, and promoting a unique perspective on the world. It is best learned initially with the guidance of a qualified yoga teacher.

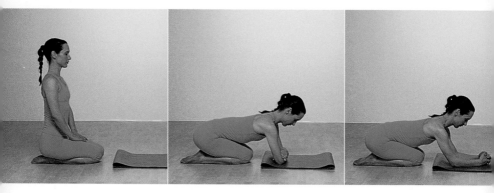

1 Kneel on the floor with your hands on your thighs. Place a folded nonslip mat in front of you. Inhale.

2 On an exhalation, bring your elbows to the mat, shoulder-distance apart. Push the them into the mat.

3 Keeping your elbows still, interlock your fingers and rest your wrists on the mat. Roll your shoulders back and down.

TAKE CARE
Avoid if you have HBP, heart disease, glaucoma, a detached retina, other problems with your eyes or ears, congestion, neck problems, if you are very overweight, or if you are menstruating.

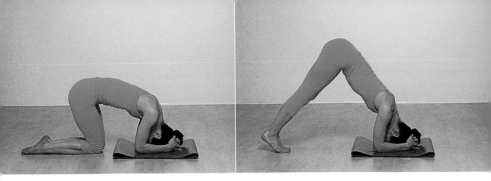

Bring the crown of your head to the floor and cradle the back of your head in the palms of your interlocked hands. Inhale.

On an exhalation, lift shoulders back and down away from your ears. Tuck toes under and straighten your legs, so you feel your weight resting now on your elbows and forearms. Lift your buttocks high.

Keeping the weight on your forearms and your shoulders away from your ears, begin to tiptoe your feet toward your head. Be aware of the shift in your center of balance as the feet come closer to your head. Sense that your spine is becoming vertical as the tailbone moves to align above the head. Breathe easily. ▶

Tip lower back slowly up to vertical

Keep shoulders lifted high away from ears

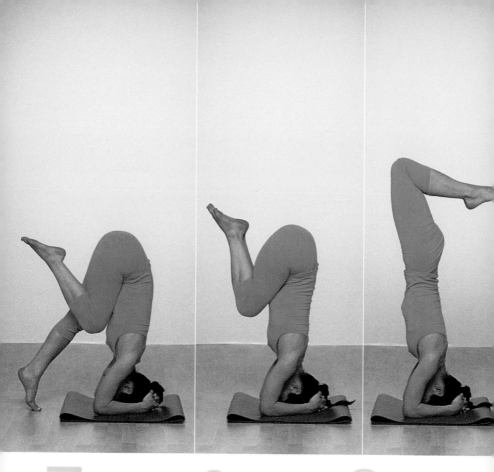

7 At the point when you feel the weight of your body shifting, pick one foot up from the floor, keeping the knee tucked in. Breathe freely like this.

8 Pick up the other foot. Stay in this position with the knees tucked in while you breathe easily and adjust yourself to the inversion.

9 When you feel confident and balanced, slowly lift the knees up, first to hip height, then above the hips. Allow the breath to flow easily.

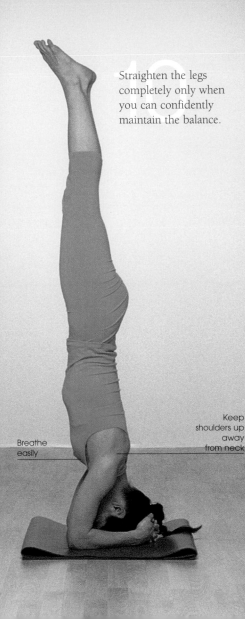

Straighten the legs completely only when you can confidently maintain the balance.

Breathe easily

Keep shoulders up away from neck

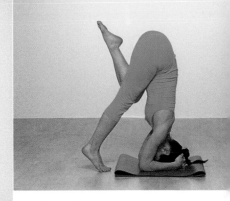

To come out of the posture, slowly tuck the knees down into the abdomen as in Step 8. Pause, then lower the feet, one at a time, to the floor.

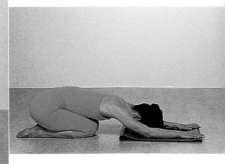

Bring the buttocks back onto the heels. Exhale completely and rest in Hare (see p.74) with the forehead on the mat.

spinal twist

Restful and refreshing, this simple twist stretches the abdominals and helps relieve stiffness caused by prolonged sitting. It also opens the chest, and promotes flexibility in the hips.

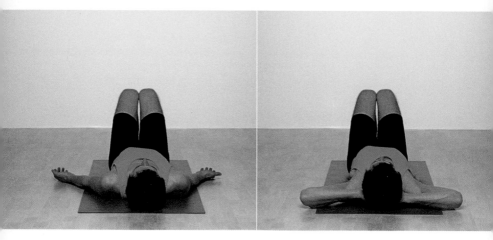

1 Lie on the floor with your knees bent and the soles of your feet flat. Keep the knees together and the back of your waist flat on the floor.

2 Clasp your hands behind the back of your head and let your elbows open out wide to the sides. Check that your chin is tucked in. Breathe into the abdomen.

On an exhalation, let your knees drop down toward the floor on the right-hand side, keeping them together as they are lowered down.

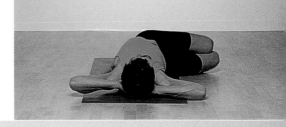

Once your knees reach the floor, turn your head to the left, breathing evenly. To come out of the pose, on an inhalation bring your head and knees back to the center. Repeat on the other side.

Let hips turn fully

Keep elbows down

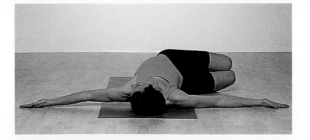

ALTERNATIVE

If your elbows do not reach the floor, take your arms out to the side at shoulder level. Feel the contact between the shoulder blades and the floor. Keep chest open.

spinal twist 2

This pose has the same benefits as Spinal Twist (see p.90), stretching the abdominals and relieving stiffness caused by prolonged sitting. It also frees blocked energy in the shoulders and hips.

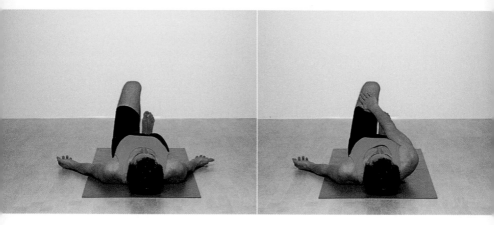

1 Lie on the floor with your legs stretched out, the knees and ankles together, and your arms stretched out to the sides, palms facing up. Bend your left knee and tuck the toes of your left foot under the back of your right knee.

2 Move your right arm across your body and place the palm of your right hand on your left thigh just above the knee. Breathe into the abdomen.

On an exhalation, allow your left knee to move across the body to drop down toward the floor. Once the knee reaches the floor, let it rest there, with your hand on top.

Turn your head to the left and breathe evenly in the pose for a few breaths. To come out of the pose, on an inhalation bring your head and left knee back to the center. Then repeat on the other side.

Let arm relax down onto floor

Let shoulder blade lift off from floor

Keep knee in contact with floor

ALTERNATIVE

To work the shoulder girdle more strongly, practice maintaining contact between the shoulder blades and the floor. This will probably mean that your knee will not reach the floor, so hold it in position with your hand.

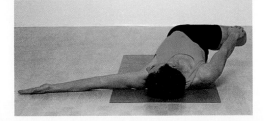

breathing
practices

The following breathing practices can be practiced on their own to improve your awareness of the breath, but they are particularly useful as preparatory practices before meditation (see p.106).

The breathing practices described here will help improve your breath awareness and encourage calmness and mental clarity. They are generally practiced after doing some yoga postures or simple stretching. Physical movement helps loosen up the body, so that it is easier to be relaxed during the breathing practices. Breath awareness is the crucial first step toward moving your attention within and learning to observe thoughts, feelings, and patterns of behavior.

Incorporating a mudra
You might like to use a mudra, or hand gesture, in conjuction with one of the breathing practices to improve its effectiveness. There are many mudras used in yoga practice. Two –

the Gesture of Consciousness and the Gesture of Knowledge – are shown on pp.104–105. They also help to remind you of the link between the individual and universal consciousness – that we are all interconnected, never unsupported.

When you are familiar with Alternate Nostril Breathing (see opposite), try visualizing the movement of the breath without using the hands whenever you need to center yourself. Called Psychic Triangle Breathing, this can be useful when you need to re-establish confidence in a public place.

Stoking the Fire (see p.96) and Shining the Skull (see p.97) are best learned with a teacher. If you have any problems, be sure to seek help.

alternate nostril breathing

Breathing through alternate nostrils has a balancing effect on the mind, body, and emotions. Begin by observing the breath and then practicing the complete breath (see p.23). Do several rounds.

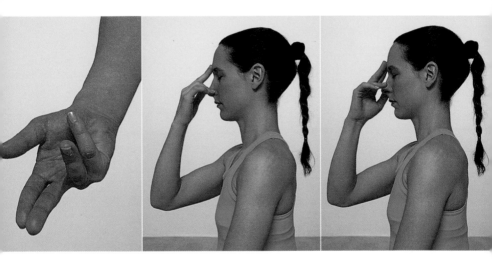

1 Sit comfortably. Lift the breastbone and relax the shoulders. Fold the little finger of the right hand into the palm. Keep the index and middle fingers straight and let the tip of the ring finger be opposite the thumb.

2 Raise your right hand to your face. Rest the index and middle fingers of the right hand between the eyebrows. Close the left nostril with your ring finger and breathe in through the right nostril.

3 Close the right nostril with the thumb and open the left. Breathe out through the left nostril, then breathe back in through it. Close the left nostril, open the right, and breathe out through that. This completes one round.

stoking the fire

This practice, which should be done on an empty stomach, develops great power in the abdominal muscles, promoting excellent digestion, increasing vitality, and helping to overcome depression and lethargy.

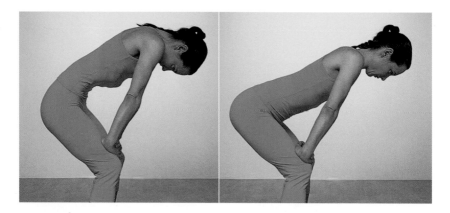

1 Stand with the feet hip-width apart. Bend the knees slightly and rest the heels of your hands on the thighs. Breathe evenly. Extend each inhalation and exhalation, so that you can feel the abdominal muscles "squeezing" the exhalation out. At the end of the next breath out, do not breathe in. Squeeze the muscles in a little tighter.

2 Release the muscles, letting the belly flop forward. Then pull the abdominal muscles sharply back in, and release them. Repeat, squeezing in and letting go of the muscles until you need to breathe in.

TAKE CARE
• If you experience dizziness or breathlessness, stop, take a break, then try more slowly and less forcefully. • Avoid if you have HBP or epilepsy, during menstruation, or if both nostrils are congested.

shining the skull

Like Stoking the Fire (see opposite), this practice should only be done on an empty stomach. It develops great power in the abdominal muscles, aids digestion, and increases vitality. Above all, it promotes clarity of mind.

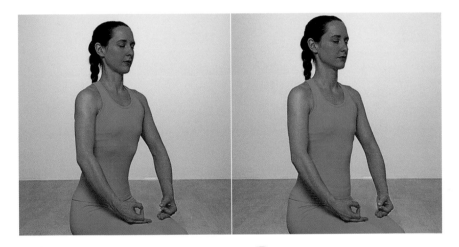

1 Kneel with the hands on the knees in the Gesture of Consciousness (see p.104). Feel the movement of the abdomen as you breathe in and out. At the end of an inhalation, draw the abdominal muscles in quickly and forcefully. This expels the air through the nose; the exhalation is felt and heard as the air leaves the nostrils.

2 Immediately allow the abdomen to release into softness, so that the inhalation happens all by itself. Repeat three to five times.

TAKE CARE
The same as for Stoking the Fire (see opposite).

humming breath

Humming breath is an antidote to stress, anger, and anxiety. It also induces a profound sense of calm, lowers blood pressure, and relieves insomnia. It strengthens the voice and promotes a relaxing inner peace.

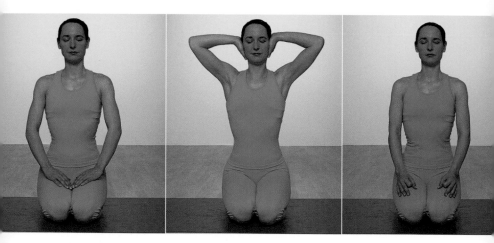

1 Sit comfortably with a straight spine in whichever of the sitting postures you prefer – Thunderbolt (see p.62) is a good basic position. Close your eyes and establish a complete breath (see p.23).

2 As you inhale, bend the elbows and draw them out wide at shoulder height. Block your ears with the heels of your hands. Keep the mouth closed, jaw relaxed, and teeth slightly apart as you breathe out, resonating a deep soft humming sound.

3 Allow the sound to fade at the end of the exhalation. Breathe normally. This is one round. Repeat five times. Keep your hands in position throughout. At the end of the last round, rest your hands in the Gesture of Knowledge (see p.105).

breath balancing

This practice promotes even breathing, aids digestion, and is a fast and effective way to center yourself.

Just a couple of minutes of breath balancing creates a calm and attentive frame of mind.

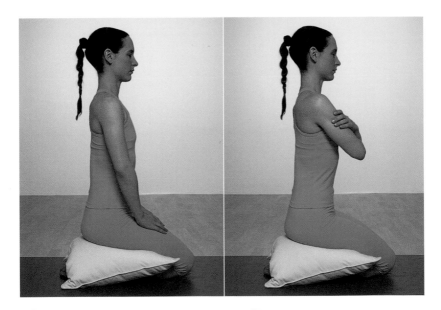

1 Sit on your heels with a straight spine. If this is uncomfortable, place a pillow between the buttocks and heels. Lower the shoulders away from the ears. With the hands resting on the thighs, watch the breath for seven rounds as you establish a complete breath (see p.23).

2 When the breath is rhythmic, tuck the right thumb high into the left armpit and the left thumb into the right armpit. Close the eyes. Be aware of a triangular pattern of breath, as the air flows into the nostrils and up the sides of the nose to the tip of the triangle between the eyebrows.

invocation of energy

Also known as "the peace gesture," this is an effective way of increasing vitality, trust, and confidence. The practice involves synchronizing the breath with arm movements. It is a symbolic giving and receiving of energy, which creates a powerful sense of tranquility and acceptance.

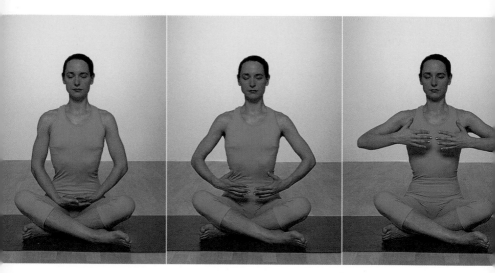

1 Sit comfortably with your legs crossed. Close your eyes. Cup your hands and rest them, palms facing upward, in your lap. Breathe evenly for three rounds.

2 As the abdomen begins to expand on the next inhalation, separate the hands and move them up to a little in front of the abdomen, tips of the fingers pointing toward each other.

3 As the ribcage begins to expand on the next inhalation, lift your hands up to just in front of your chest, until they are level with your nipples.

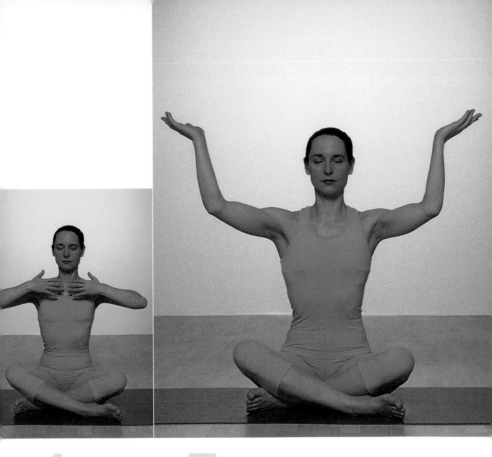

4 At the next inhalation, feel the top of your lungs expand as you raise your hands up to the level of the collarbones.

5 Hold your breath in your lungs as you open out your arms and turn your palms face up. Remain in this position for as long as you can comfortably retain the breath. On the exhalation, gradually move the hands back down to the lap. Relax and breathe normally.

concentration
practices

Concentration practices develop mental focus, which is one of the key foundations of self-confidence. They also improve memory and can relieve anxiety, depression, and insomnia.

concentrated gazing

This practice begins by providing an external point of focus, and then shifts the attention to the after-image, which appears in the mind's eye. Withdrawing your attention to the internal world is a crucial step in acquiring the attentive self-awareness and quiet interior focus necessary to building self-esteem.

Use a comfortable seated position, such as Thunderbolt (see p.62), and position a candle at arm's length in front of you so that its flame will be

precisely at eye level. With your head, neck, and spine aligned, place your hands in the Gesture of Knowledge (see p.105). Establish a rhythmic complete breath (see p.23) as you relax in your chosen seated posture.

Gradually increase the length of time you can gaze at the candle without blinking. Take it easy, and never strain the eyes. If you find that you become agitated by the rapidity or the nature of the thoughts and images passing through your mind, stop the practice and seek advice from a yoga teacher who has experience of its effects.

Developing mental focus and concentration takes time and patience, so, as you notice different thoughts or emotions, gently redirect your attention back to the object of your gaze.

PRACTICAL MATTERS
• Remove eyeglasses or contact lenses before starting the practice.
• Make sure the room is not drafty; otherwise, the flame of the candle will flicker and be distracting.

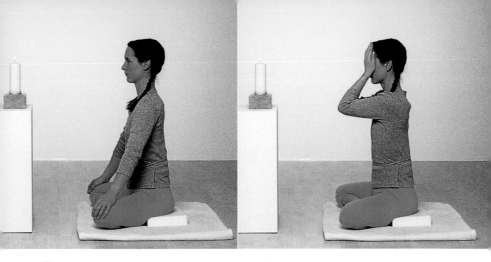

1 Let your gaze come to rest steadily on the flame at the tip of the candle wick. Allow your eyes to fix their gaze on this point without blinking or moving. Focus the awareness so completely on the flame that you are no longer consciously aware of your physical body.

Keep your gaze steady for as long as you can. When the eyes start to water or feel tired, gently close them. With the eyes closed, focus on the after-image of the candle flame that appears in the space in front of the closed eyes. Try to keep that image in place for as long as possible.

When the image begins to fade, open the eyes and look at the candle again. Keep the gaze focused for as long as you can, then close the eyes, focusing on the after-image of the candle. Repeat three or four times.

2 Rub your palms together vigorously until they feel warm, and cup the palms over your eyes. Feel the heat from the hands bathing the eyelids. Keeping the palms in place, open your eyes and look into the darkness within your cupped hands. When you are ready, lower your hands from your face.

TAKE CARE

• If you have epilepsy, do not focus on a candle flame, but instead use a fixed point, or an object or image of your choice.
• If you have severe eyestrain, myopia, astigmatism, or cataracts, use a black dot instead of a flame.
• If it is hard to focus on the flame at arm's length (because you are near- or far-sighted, for example), choose a distance at which you can focus easily, without straining the eyes.

using mudras

Mudras are traditional hand gestures that help you to center yourself. They help you quieten when you are feeling stressed, promoting a calm, meditative state of mind in which trust can be developed.

gesture of consciousness

Sitting cross-legged with your eyes closed, rest the backs of the hands on the knees or thighs, with the palms up. Bring the tip of each index finger to touch the tip of the thumb. Allow the rest of the fingers to be straight, but also relaxed and slightly apart from each other. Alternatively, tuck the tip of each index finger into the root of the thumb. You can also practice this mudra kneeling in Thunderbolt pose (see p.62).

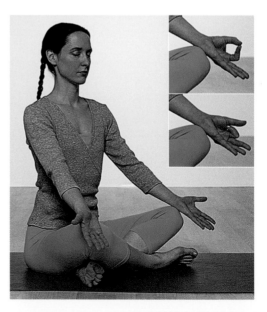

gesture of knowledge

Sitting with legs crossed (or in Thunderbolt – see p.62) and eyes closed, rest the palms of the hands on the knees or the thighs. Bring the tip of the index finger to touch the tip of the thumb. Alternatively, tuck the tip of each index finger into the root of the thumb. Let the rest of the fingers be straight but still, relaxed and slightly apart from one another. This is a more inward-looking gesture than the Gesture of Consciousness, and is suitable for deeper exploration of your attitudes and beliefs.

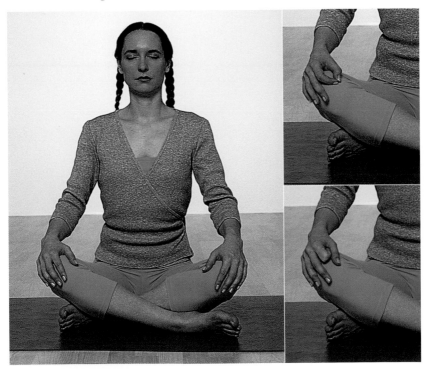

meditation

Meditation is a simple but profound practice that can bring about a state of focused attention and peace. Practiced often, it can teach you to observe and understand your thoughts and emotions.

inner silence meditation

This meditation practice takes about 15 minutes to complete. Sit in a comfortable position and close your eyes. Establish a Full Yogic Breath (see p.23). Rest your hands in the Gesture of Consciousness (see p.104).

PRACTICAL MATTERS
• Choose a time when you are certain that you will remain undisturbed for at least 15 minutes.
• Choose a room (or space outside) that is quiet, uncluttered, and not cold or drafty.
• Choose a posture – sitting in a chair, or sitting or kneeling on the floor – that you will be able to sustain easily for some time.

Let your awareness be with the sense of hearing. Listen to all the sounds. Start by bringing your attention to the loudest, then gradually draw the focus of your awareness in closer until you attend only to the quietest, closest sounds. Be aware of the sound of your own breath as it comes in and goes out.

Now shift the focus of your attention to the sense of touch. Become aware of the sensation of the breath passing into and out of the nostrils. Feel the cooler air coming in and the warmer air going out. Be aware of the different textures and temperatures that you can detect through the sense of touch. Sense if there is any difference between what you can feel on covered and uncovered skin. Then return to feeling the passage of air in the nose.

Now give your full attention to the sense of smell. Be aware of any odors and aromas around you. Then shift your attention to the sense of taste. Be aware of the tongue inside the mouth. Notice if there are sweet, salty, bitter, hot, or astringent tastes. Give the sense of taste full attention.

Now focus your attention on the sense of sight. Look into the closed eyelids and be aware of whatever you may see there. Are there any colors or shapes? Are there patterns, or movement? Just blackness?

Now spend a few moments simply watching the patterns of your own thoughts as they arise and pass away. Sit and wait for the first thought, watch it until it passes away, and then wait for the next thought to arrive. Do not get caught up with your thoughts or try to follow them.

After a little while, return your attention to the sense of hearing, and become aware of the intimate sound

of your own breath. Allow that breath to get a little louder, and use the sound of that breath as a bridge back to becoming aware of other sounds in the room. Then widen your awareness until you are aware of sounds out in the wider world. When you are ready, open your eyes.

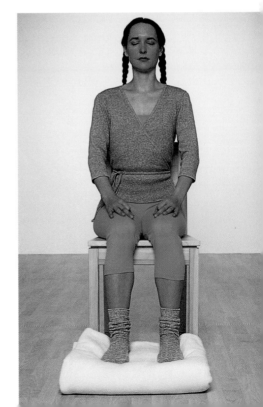

relaxation

Relaxing at the end of a yoga session gives the body and mind a chance to absorb the benefits of your practice. Set aside 20 minutes and follow the Deep Relaxation practice described below.

deep relaxation

This is a shortened version of one of the most powerful systematic approaches to profound relaxation. The Sanskrit for this practice is *yoga nidra* with *sankalpa*, which translates as "yogic sleep with affirmation." In fact, it is only the body that sleeps while the mind remains alert.

Lie on the floor in Corpse pose (see opposite). Close your eyes and establish 11 rounds of the complete breath (see p.23). Feel yourself settling the body into a state of stillness. Become aware of the points of contact between body and floor.

Make a resolve to let the body take deep rest, while the mind remains alert and attentive. Then prepare to carry the mental attention around the body, visiting each part of the body in turn, as if the light of the mind's attention were to come to shine briefly on each body part.

Keeping absolutely still, now bring the mental attention to touch each part of your body in turn. Choose a circuit that you can remember and that covers every part of the body. Try scanning down from top to bottom, or working clockwise around the body, or from the edges to the center.

When you have touched each part of the body in turn with your mental attention, bring the focus of your awareness back to the rhythm of the complete breath. Count 27 rounds of this, beginning at 27, and counting down to zero. If you lose count, start again.

When you get to the end of the last round of the complete breath, return to the resolve to let the body take deep rest, while the mind remains alert and attentive. Sense that the body is fully rested, and that the mind is alert and attentive. Then let your breath get a little noisier, until you can hear it clearly. Use the sound of the breath as the bridge back to a more everyday state of awareness. Stretch out through the fingers and toes, the hands and feet. Then stretch out through the whole body, roll over and sit up. When you feel ready, open your eyes.

Adding an affirmation

Once your are familiar with the sequence, you may want to make your own affirmation. Choose a simple, short, and positive statement about a direction you would like your life to take. Choose carefully, and make sure that you are happy with the affirmation before you work with it. When you feel you have the right affirmation, use it at the start and end of the relaxation practice.

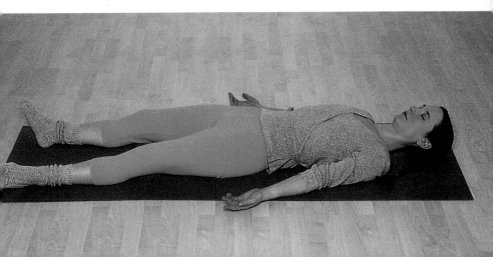

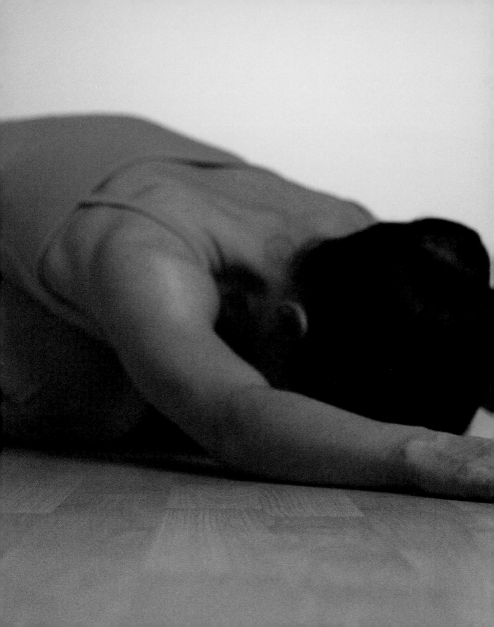

| part **3**

programs

The following seven programs will help boost your confidence in a variety of situations: before an exam or interview, during change and disruption, at times of self-doubt, when feeling panicky, when facing a challenge, and when you need to develop your self-worth.

① pre-interview
boost

Remaining confident and relaxed during an interview can be a challenge. This sequence, practiced before you set out for the interview, develops the energy and focus to approach your meeting positively. The final two practices can also be repeated on the way to the interview to maintain confidence and clarity of focus.

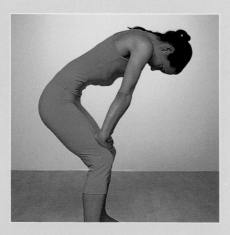

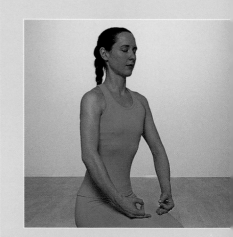

① Stoking the Fire (see p.96)

② Shining the Skull (see p.97)

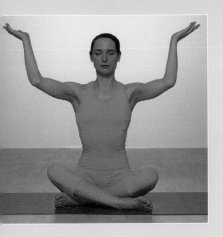

3 Invocation of Energy (see pp.100–101)

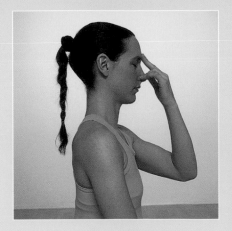

4 Alternate Nostril Breathing (see p.95)

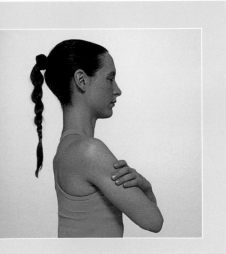

5 Breath Balancing (see p.99)

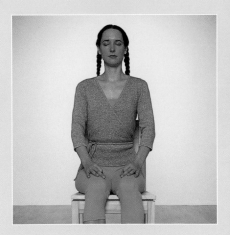

6 Inner Silence Meditation (see pp.106–107)

2 in times of change

This sequence enhances your ability to adapt to changes in all aspects of life. To deepen the effect, practice the complete breath (see p.23) in Reverse Corpse, and abdominal breathing (see p.23) in Hare. Use a focused gaze during Snake and Triangle. Complete the program with a period of Inner Silence Meditation (see p.106).

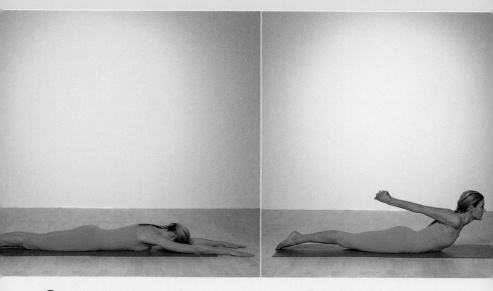

1 Reverse Corpse (see p.54)

2 Snake (see pp.52–53)

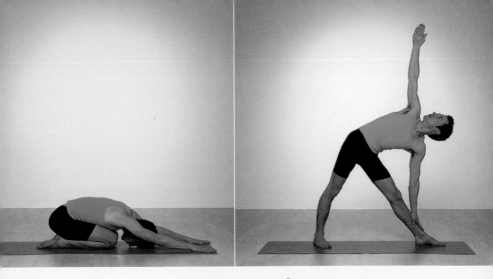

3 Hare (see pp.74–75)

4 Triangle (see pp.38–39)

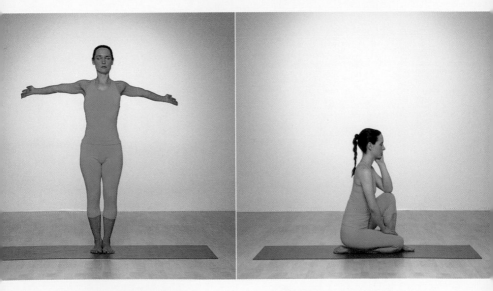

5 Arm Stretch 3 (see p.26)

6 Philosopher (see pp.64–65)

③ at low
moments

If you feel depressed, this program can help shift blocked energy, lift your spirits, and restore self-esteem. Begin with a few rounds of Stoking the Fire (see p.96). Allow the complete breath (see p.23) to flow through the Dancer, Tree, and Camel. Conclude with a stabilizing two minutes of Alternate Nostril Breathing (see p.95).

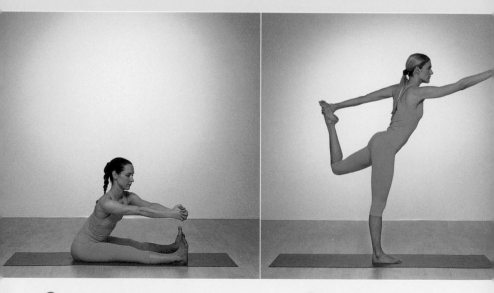

❶ Stirring the Pot (see pp.32–33)   **❷ Dancer** (see pp.42–43)

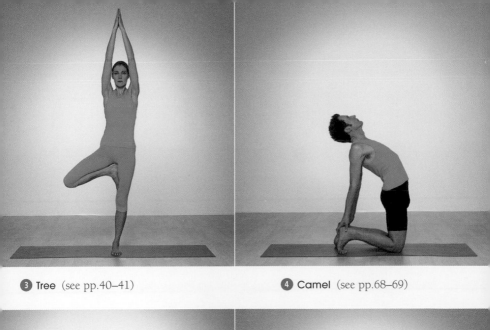

3 Tree (see pp.40–41)

4 Camel (see pp.68–69)

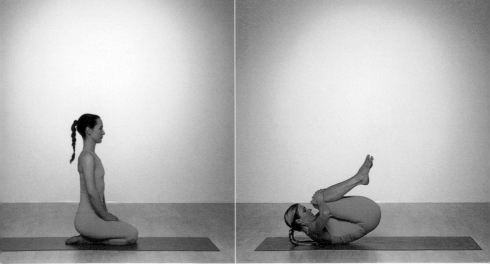

5 Thunderbolt (see pp.62–63)

6 Yogic Rock and Roll (see p.29)

(4) for balance &
understanding

A balancing yoga program can help when your tolerance is challenged. Start with two minutes of the complete breath (see p.23). Then move through the postures, focusing on the breath. Complete the program with 27 rounds of Breath Balancing (see p.99) in Thunderbolt (see p.62), followed by Deep Relaxation (see p.108).

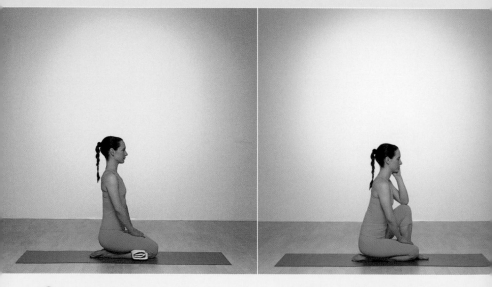

1 Thunderbolt (see pp.62–63)

2 Philosopher (see pp.64–65)

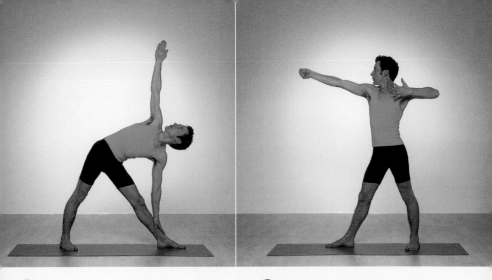

3 Triangle (see pp.38–39)

4 Bow and Arrow (see pp.36–37)

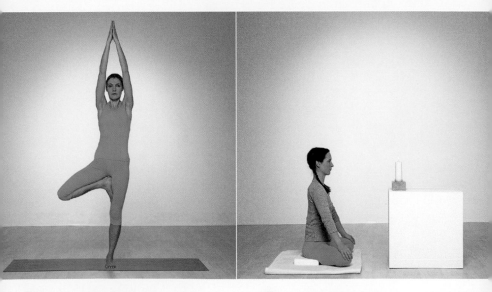

5 Tree (see pp.40–41)

6 Concentrated Gazing (see pp.102–103)

5 for
stability & ease

This sequence brings the focus within, developing easeful self-acceptance. Begin with 11 rounds of the complete breath (see p.23) in Thunderbolt. Then hold each posture for at least seven abdominal breaths (see p.23). Complete the program with 11 rounds of Humming Breath (see p.98), followed by Deep Relaxation (see p.108).

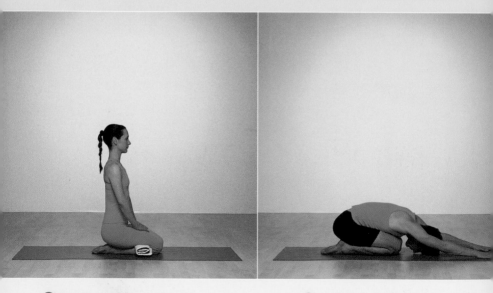

1 Thunderbolt (see pp.62–63)   **2** Hare (see pp.74–75)

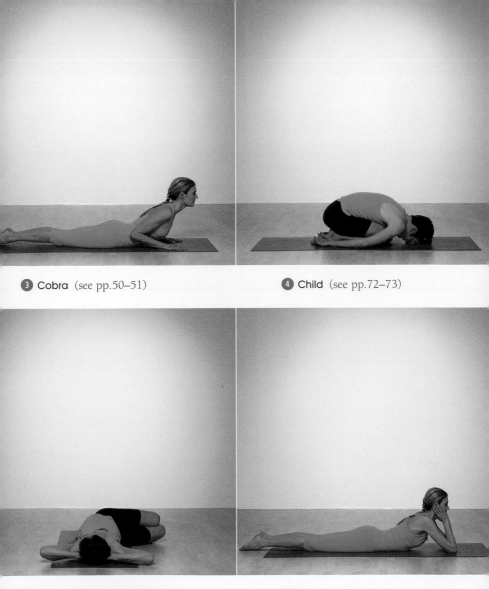

3 Cobra (see pp.50–51)

4 Child (see pp.72–73)

5 Spinal Twist (see pp.90–91)

6 Resting Crocodile (see pp.54–55)

6 for
courage

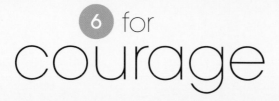

This program promotes strength and self-confidence to develop courage. Begin with seven rounds of the complete breath (see p.23). After Boat, do another 11 complete breaths before continuing with the postures. Conclude by quiet sitting in Thunderbolt (see p.62) and five rounds of Invocation of Energy (see p.100).

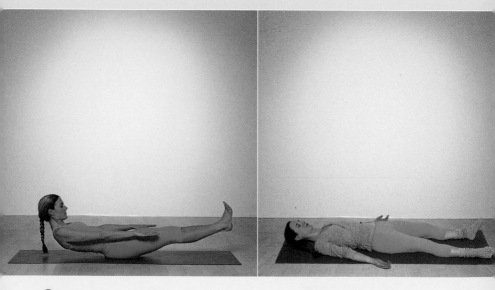

1 **Boat** (see pp.44–45)

2 **Corpse** (see p.109)

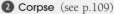

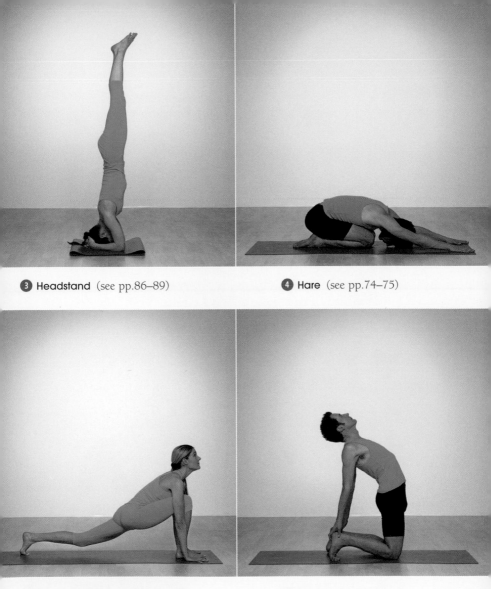

3 Headstand (see pp.86–89)

4 Hare (see pp.74–75)

5 Lunge Warrior (see pp.48–49)

6 Camel (see pp.68–69)

⑦ to develop
self-worth

This program fosters compassionate self-acceptance and focused conviction. Take 11 rounds of the complete breath (see p.23) before you begin the postures, and another seven rounds after Boat. At the end of the program, do Inner Silence Meditation (see p.106), followed by Deep Relaxation (see p.108), using an affirmation.

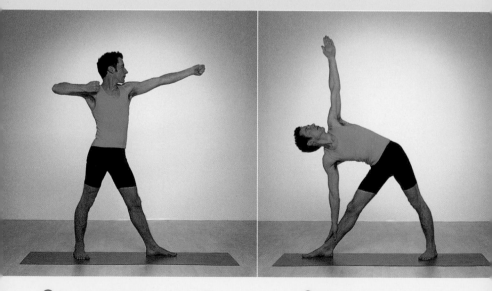

① **Bow and Arrow** (see pp.36–37)

② **Triangle** (see pp.38–39)

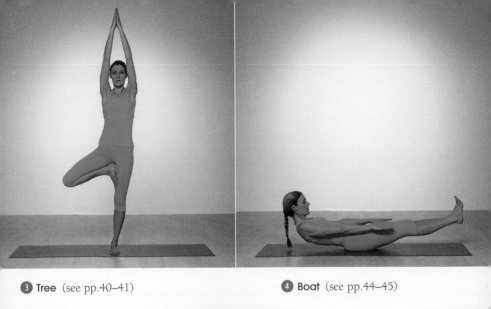

3 Tree (see pp.40–41)

4 Boat (see pp.44–45)

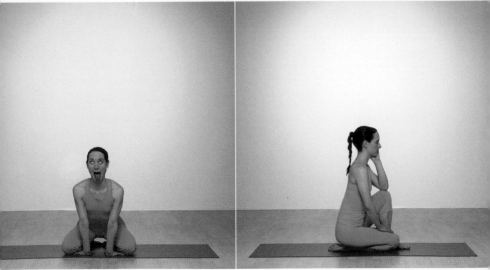

5 Roaring Lion (see pp.66–67)

6 Philosopher (see pp.64–65)

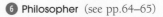

Index

Useful organizations

www.yogasite.com
A general source of information on yoga, with good links, and a teachers' directory covering the United States, Canada, Australia, and other countries.

THE BRITISH WHEEL OF YOGA
Tel: 01529 306851;
Website: www.bwy.org.uk
Provides information on classes, yoga organizations, and events in the UK.

www.yogafinder.com
A directory listing yoga teachers, organizations, and events in the United States and other countries.

THE YOGA THERAPY CENTRE
Tel: 020 7869 3040;
Website: www.yogatherapy.org
The Yoga Biomedical Trust's center for yoga therapy, general yoga classes, workshops and training.

Acknowledgments

AUTHOR'S ACKNOWLEDGMENTS
Thanks to my mother, for teaching me confidence and showing me yoga at the age of four. Gratitude for the patience of my husband and sons. Dedicated to the living legacies of all Swami Sivananda's disciples who shine the light of yoga throughout the world, especially Paramahamsa Satyananda Saraswati. Om Namaya Shiva.

PUBLISHER'S ACKNOWLEDGMENTS
Thanks to Catherine MacKenzie for design assistance; Helen Ridge, Jane Simmonds, and Angela Wilkes for editorial assistance; Dorothy Frame for indexing; Katy Wall for jacket design; and Anna Bedewell for additional picture research.

Models: Lee Hamblin, Kelly Smith–Beaney, Cate Williams
Photographer's Assistant: Nick Rayment
Hair and Make-up: Hitoko Honbu (represented by Hers) **Studio:** Air Studios Ltd

Yoga mats: Hugger Mugger Yoga Products, 12 Roseneath Place, Edinburgh EH9 1JB. **Tel**: 44 (0) 131 221 9977; **Fax**: 44 (0) 131 2291 9112; **Website**: www.yoga.co.uk; **email**: info @huggermugger.co.uk
In the US, these mats can be obtained from: Hugger Mugger Products, 3937 SO 500 W, Salt Lake City, Utah 84123. **Tel**: 800 473 4888; **Fax**: 801 268 2629; **Website**: www.huggermugger.com
Yoga props: Yoga Matters, 42 Priory Road, London N8 7EX. **Tel**: 44 (0) 20 8348 1203; **Website**: www.yogamatters.co.uk; **email**: enquiries@yogamatters.co.uk

PICTURE CREDITS
The publisher would like to thank the following for their kind permission to reproduce their photographs.
7: Photonica/Mats Widen; 12: Getty Images/Justin Pumfrey; 16: Getty Images/Anthony Marsland. All other images © Dorling Kindersley. For further information see: www.dkimages.com